4-19-98

after being guided by
spirit to this Yoga,
I decided to by this book
since I desire a clearer
understanding of their concepts
and beliefs. Ultimately I find
they are the same as mine
or the ~~same~~ ones thing
I myself am striving 4.

God Speed

ॐ Om

Shanti

Cause God said let there
Be light..

Seek ye 1st the Kingdom of
heaven and all shall Be
added unto you

Om shanti

"The essays in this book are inspired meditations on the great spiritual themes of alienation, action, suffering, self-sacrifice, non-duality, and liberation. More than being wise commentaries on spiritual life, they also have a poetic and mantric quality that draws the reader into the meditative state. This is a highly practical book."

- **GEORG FEUERSTEIN, Ph.D.**, author of *Encyclopedic Dictionary of Yoga*; *Holy Madness*; *Yoga, the Technology of Ecstasy*, etc.

"*Ways of Yoga* is a unique book that describes the path to human liberation in a simple style. Using both a conversational and meditational tone, the book describes joyful freedom in action, change, sacrifice, work, love and relationship.

- ***HINDUISM TODAY***

"*Ways of Yoga* administers a curative shock. Christian readers will learn God doesn't do it all; Buddhist readers will learn desire doesn't spoil it all; New Age readers will learn pain doesn't ruin it all. In this book, Gurāṇi Añjali marvelously teaches the mind/body through the body (the exercises) and the mind (the meditations). I can testify to her many *siddhi*."

- **ROBERT MAGLIOLA**, Distinguished Chair Professor, the Graduate School, National Taiwan University, author of *Derrida on the Mend*, etc.

". . . to help renew a union with the light in our own lives. . ."

- ***YOGA JOURNAL***

"This book introduces the reader into new ways of seeing and practicing the Yoga tradition. Based on meditations spoken by Gurāṇi Añjali at her Ashram in Amityville, New York, *Ways of Yoga* offers a series of reflections and meditation exercises that show how Yoga can speak directly to the issues of contemporary life. Like Swami Vivekananda, she uses stories and quotations from sacred texts to illustrate her teachings. Additionally, this volume includes guided meditations that can be practiced to gain deeper insight into yogic experience. I highly recommend this book for persons seeking to learn more about this ancient path."

-**CHRISTOPHER CHAPPLE, Ph.D.**, Associate Professor of Theology, Loyola Marymount University, author of *Karma and Creativity* and *Yoga Sutras of Patañjali*, etc.

Ways of Yoga is a must read for Yoga students. . . The meditations themselves are practical and accessible. . . ."

-**YOGA INTERNATIONAL**

"In that momentary hesitation before writing these words, the intimate feel of this text wins through. Gurāṇi Añjali's conversational tone evokes the flow of a cool stream on a hot day - one look and one wants to get in. After entering, one finds the traditional practice of Vedic sacrifice set in a contemporary context and the withdrawal of Upanishadic wisdom nuanced for the modern American 'loner'. . . . Her stress on sacrifice, interdependence, and self-confrontation inculcate a spirit of liberation in discipline. She espies a selfless work for us in serving others - especially our fellow creatures on this earth. Her charm is her subtle ability to evoke the joy in the work!"

- **JOHN GRIM, Ph.D.**, Associate Professor, Dept. of Religion, Bucknell University.

WAYS OF YOGA

by

GURĀṆI AÑJALI

With an Introduction by

Yogi Ananda Virāj

Vajra Printing and Publishing
of Yoga Anand Ashram

First Edition 1993

Published by:
Vajra Printing & Publishing of Y.A.A.
49 Forrest Place
Amityville, NY 11701

These essays are based on meditations held at Yoga Anand Ashram, Amityville, New York. "The Yoga of Action" was first published in *Moksha Journal*, Volume I, Number 2 (1984) and is reprinted here with permission.

The Introduction by Yogi Ananda Virāj, copyright 1984 by Yoga Anand Ashram, is reprinted here in revised form with permission.

Printed in the United States of America

Library of Congress Cataloging in Publication Data

Añjali, Gurāni
Ways of Yoga / by Gurāṇi Añjali:
with an introduciton by Yogi Ananda Virāj
- First Edition

p. cm.
Includes index.
1. Yoga. I. Title.
BL 1238.52.A55 1993 294.5'43 --dc20 CIP 90-72045
ISBN 0-933989-01-6 : $ 10.95 softcover

10 9 8 7 6 5 4 3 2

Cover Art Design by Gurāṇi Añjali

Dedicated

to the memory of my father

Śṛī Inti Gurumūrti

Acknowledgements

I thank all members of Yoga Anand Ashram for supporting me in the undertaking of this book.

My deep gratitude goes to Yogi Ananda Virāj for his pleasurable conversations which provoked a stimulus and for his continuous editing and final editing. My gratitude and special thanks to Professor Christopher Chapple and his wife Maureen for their sincere efforts and kind thoughts, particularly at the onset of this undertaking. My warmest gratitude goes to Rocco Lo Bosco who worked on editing long and patiently from start to finish. My gratitude also goes to Yogi Ananda Satyam, who diligently worked on editing and promotion. My sincere thanks goes to Dolores Burns, Secretary of Yoga Anand Ashram, for computer and typing work. Without her this book would be non-existent. Many thanks to Glenn James of Vajra Printing & Publishing, and sincere thanks to his wife Teresa for helping along.

Many thanks to William Bilodeau, Alan Buehler, Roy Mitchell, Steve Crimi, Loretta Quintano, Nancy Caruso and many thanks to Debra Nord for art work, and to Frances Keaveny for photography.

TABLE OF CONTENTS

TABLE OF CONTENTS

INTRODUCTION

by Yogi Ananda Virāj

Him with fair wings though only One,
poets shape, with songs,
in many forms.
Ṛg Veda 10.114.5

It is an honor for me to help establish an approach to the reflections and meditation exercises of Guraṇi Añjali. From my point of view these stem from the depths of her profound and yet ordinary vision. As I have witnessed her life for over seventeen years she has demonstrated a stability which I can only characterize as enlightened. She carries on the business of everydayness with a subtle strength that displays her immersion in wisdom and compassion. Because of the selfless attitude she lives, she remains open to quiet revelations. It is these revelations which, through her concern for others, give rise to this book. I deeply hope that this introduction does justice to its origin.

At first glance the writings contained herein might seem to demand more explanation, and to some extent that is what we will be providing. But given a closer look, and more importantly a try, something unusual begins to emerge: these insights defy any single explanation.There is a simple explanation for this, however, and that is that above all else these reflections and meditation exercises affect the body. At this point what has been said may appear to be trivial. Of course exercises exercise the body, at least those that employ body movements. However, this is not what we mean by exercise of the body.

First let us establish what we mean by the "body." From a Yogic point of view our ordinary commonsense world is a world comprised of things, entities, persons, places; in short, discreteness. The language we use to describe such a world is the language of *prakṛti*. *Prakṛti*, through its functionaries the three *guṇas*, constructs a lived world in which understanding *(buddhi)*, individuality *(ahaṃkāra)*, conceptuality (*manas* or mind), and sense organs give rise to sensations, perception, personality, objects, relations, feelings, attachments, aversions, etc. In other words, *prakṛti* composes our normal body-world-view. However, life within this world-view is often replete with the sorrow that arises from challenges to this world-view. Conflicts of interest on personal, social, ideological and religious grounds often land us in confusion and turmoil, frequently generating the need to question the view. Basically, two forms of questioning arise: the first is a superficial form and the second a radical form. The result of the first is often compromise, a bending of the view simply to get along in an environment of conflict. The aim of the second is to bring to the surface the assumptions or determinations which structure the world-view in question. This is undertaken to better understand "myself" and/or "my world" in the hope that "I" will be prepared to cope with life and escape sorrow. What this second form of inquiry ignores, however, is that life itself is a product of view and no amount of questioning, analysis or explanation is radical enough to get at the "root." In other words, the images or fundamental assumptions which lie in the understanding *(buddhi)* and give rise to the sense of individuality *(ahaṃkāra)*, sensation (body) and world are too deep, too incarnate, to reveal themselves to cognition in such a way as to free us from them. What is required is experience.

Given that our living mind-body-world is structured according to deeply-rooted images, the Yogic task is to transcend these images, thereby transcending the narrow world-view dogmatically held and repeatedly threatened. In short, Yoga asks that we change the body. This change is accomplished, in view of the foregoing, by a suspension of the operations of root-imagery. We seek to suspend the operations of *prakṛti*. This brings us to the notion of the return.

Traditional Yoga practice (*sādhana*) usually takes the form of a "withdrawal." From our so-called Western perspective this word bears negative connotations, but for the time being I ask that you suspend judgement until we have seen what "Yogic" withdrawal entails and produces. The Yogic withdrawal is refocusing of attention. Given that the body-world shaped by root-imagery culminates in objects or perceived things, we begin by shifting our attention from those things to progressively more subtle constructions on a more "interior" plane. To accomplish this reversal, possessiveness, theft, greed, etc., are weakened through various ethical practices. As our attachments and aversions are reduced, we grow less committed to the body-world-view that gave rise to sorrow. Eventually our practice takes the form of meditation techniques which aim at the suspension of the view of an objective world and hence a return or retrieval of "the world" itself. However, even at these subtle stages the feeling of individuality and cognitive activity are active. If these latter are not also suspended, a reversal of the reversal will take place and once again attachments, aversions and sorrows will multiply. Eventually, with ardent practice, cognition and personality are also suspended and the "liberating experience" will ensue. This brings us to the other Yogic language, the language of *puruṣa* .

The language of *puruṣa* seeks to describe the pure consciousness at the heart of experience. *Puruṣa* is undivided awareness which animates the movements of *prakṛti*, rendering them experience. When *prakṛti* has ceased to unfold herself as the manifest order and has returned to her original condition of wholeness as the unmanifest, consciousness is revealed to be unlimited, pervading the totality. The body becomes whole and fully conscious. The return to this conscious body totality is termed *pratiprasava*, a return to the origin. This vision is a movement of body to complete incarnation. The body-feel opens to conform to this holistic knowledge, drawing itself into an integrity which momentarily obliterates all discreteness."The world becomes flesh," in total. It is a harmony wherein each part is the whole and no part is differentiated from the whole. It is a vision in which all things are resolved, taking their proper places in a "cosmic" unity. It is the experience of the One.

The practice of concentration in Yoga does just that. It concentrates all that was dispersed as body-world into a flash of totality, a vision of wholeness. In Ṛg Vedic terms this was known as the *ṛtu*, rendered by Antonio deNicolás as "the instant-moment of total presence."[1] However, as deNicolás stresses, this *ṛtu* is concomitant with re-emergence. Manifestation yearns only for return and the One yearns only for manifestation as new or different body-worlds. The suspension of the operation of *prakṛti* as root-images giving rise to bodies and worlds promotes a vision which is the source of them all. The One, or the Father, is parented by the Son. Understanding *(buddhi)* which mediates or filters this wholeness, making it accessible to the claim of individuality *(ahaṃkāra)*, now turns a backward glance to the One from which it derives the knowledge that generates the partial visions of mortals. *Buddhi* can, after the vision, manifest and nourish body-worlds which, through faith, "count on" the One. The conflict and confusion that marked the pre-vision personality can now be overcome as long as one lives and acts with a devotion to unity and wholeness. Truth becomes a living in the light of "divine harmony" and "the world" becomes one among the many possible worlds, no one order seeking dominance over another. In the body's attempt to reach the dimensions of the totality the *ṛtu* is born. In the One's urge to manifest itself the *ṛtu* gives birth to bodies. This reciprocity is the very stuff of human dignity and survival.

The experience of oneness is known in Yogic terms as *kaivalyaṃ*, translated as isolation or absolute unity. It is also known as the seer's own form *(draṣṭuḥ sva-rūpa)* (Yoga Sūtra I:3). The seer is the *puruṣa* as consciousness. Its form is the body's conformance to the dimensions of the *puruṣa*. *Kaivalyaṃ* is attained when the luminosity (*sattva-guṇa*) of *prakṛti* achieves parity, in terms of purity, with *puruṣa* (*sattva-puruṣayoḥ śuddhi-sāmye kaivalyaṃ*, Yoga Sūtra III.55).

Again, once *kaivalyaṃ* is achieved the world(s) re-emerge anew. However, now one realizes the origin of life and a different "way" of life is born. The totality descends into the *prakṛtic* realm through and in our everyday actions. By the cultivation of clarity (*sattva*), actions are undertaken without the burden of attachments and aversions. Through a *sattvic* outlook actions are performed by the totality; no one "feature" of the whole is given priority. Each "item" constituting the action is viewed, non-reflectively, as "containing" the totality. Substances, conceived of as having an independent nature, are no longer evident. What we find are things not as isolated entities but as "functions" which are not differentiated from the holistic awareness organizing the action. Therefore actions become efficient, both personally and socially, because the knowledge organizing the action is granted unhindered incarnation in a sattvic openness. In contrast, an outlook laden with desire for the results of action *(rajas guṇa)*, one emphasizing an agent who performs the action *(ahaṃkāra)*, is characterized by undue reflective activity inhibiting the move to satisfactory incarnations. It is only through the sattvic vision of homogeneity that the fabric of knowledge *(jñāna)* which unites all things in harmonious efficiency is allowed to functionally incarnate. In this instance we become instruments of knowledge, "doing the will of the Father," rather than agents of action "doing *our own* thing." The omniscience of the "Lord" *(Īśvara)* is to be counted on: "... do not worry about what you are to say; when the time comes, the words you need will be given you; for it is not you who will be speaking: it will be the Spirit of your Father speaking in you" (Matthew 10.19-20).

Recalling now our cautionary statement regarding Yogic "withdrawal," we see that the withdrawal yogis have in mind is one which leads both backward and forward. The return is concomitant with re-emergence; the end is the beginning, "I am the first and I am the last, and there is no god but me" (Isaiah 44.6).

Having been led inside of Yogic thought and language we can now proceed to give an account of the Yogic intentions of the exercises of Gurāṇi Añjali.

We have noted that the exercises exercise the body. This exercise of body is no trivial physical manipulation but a radical shifting of perspective and therefore a change of body, a reincarnation. However, there is one essential point that needs emphasis: the exercises of Gurāṇi Añjali deviate from tradition in one significant sense; they seek to afford the executor a provisional glimpse into the One. These exercises are not to be uncritically accepted as practice. Practice implies repetition, repeated performance, systematic application. The exercises can be done by practitioners and by non-practitioners alike. However, a non-practitioner can be afforded as much of a glimpse as a practitioner. On the other hand, the practitioner may be able to better exploit the exercises; that is, the prior training better prepares the body to accept the totality offered in the glimpse. Such acceptance may or may not be complete, but either way practice may better prepare the way for the vision.

As a way into the exercises we will select one which will serve as a model for understanding the rest. The exercise is called "Directions," found following this introduction. The student is asked by the guide to stand and "face" north, then turn east, south and west. This bodily orientation to the directions is repeated anywhere from three to five times, changing the order of the directions each time. The momentum is increased with each set of the four cardinal points. The incarnation of the commands now reaches an accelerated pitch that becomes the condition necessary for the issuance of the final command: "Face yourself!" The incongruity of cardinal points and self is conceptually obvious. However, the body has become sensitized to directional orientation with only minor or secondary disorientation occurring with the changing order of the cardinal points. But even this minor disorientation serves to prepare the body to "leap," if you will, beyond its felt boundaries. The final entreaty, *face yourself*, is so incarnationally incongruous that a shock is felt which, given optimal conditions, catapults one into the totality. "Where do I look for the self?" The combination of orientation via cardinal points, the *prakṛtic* or bodily move to incarnate the commands, and the acceleration of the embodiment process works to condense the construction and deconstruction of body-worlds into an intensity that sets the stage for the final breakthrough. Self is without spatial, or for that matter temporal, reference. The anticipation of the command to spatial reference, so counted on by the body, is disrupted, yet the command "face yourself" remains as if to draw the body inwards to concentrate itself in the whole. This is the moment of the *ṛtu*.

For some an authentic glimpse of the *puruṣa* occurs. Others may sense an inchoate shock which defies explanation. That is itself a glimpse of sorts. The main thing is that one be brought to experience. A momentary suspension of cognitive orientation may be enough to incite interest in going further along the way to complete incarnation. It is at this point that we can appreciate the distinction made earlier between the exercises and practice. It was stated that the glimpse afforded would be a "provisional" one. Shock can be of value; however, it is only through the cultivation of a *sattvic* or clear outlook that one can learn to accommodate the One in terms of both entering into the vision and living out the vision through effective action. Also, we can now appreciate Gurāṇi Añjali's deviation from traditional modes of "practice" in inventing these exercises. Her concern that people enter into the way of practice (*sādhana*) prompted her to seek a means whereby people could "in the twinkling of an eye" catch a glimpse of the goal and source of the Yogic way of life.

As is only obvious, some will pursue the vision and others will not. Some may read this introduction and try the exercises, some will not. My hope is that this introduction actually "leads within" to that great interior of which life is made. Negatively speaking, I hope that this examination does not defeat the purpose of the exercises by rationalizing them, denying their students access to the spontaneity they aim to release. This introduction was in no way meant to serve as a concession to the "imperialist demands" of Western rationality that all experience be reduced to the manageable limits of a theory about experience. The fullness of human life is only realized when, through our direct experience, we align ourselves with the interests of the One.

1. Antonio T. de Nicolás, *Mediations Through The Ṛg Veda* (New York: Nicolas Hayes Ltd.,1976)

MEDITATION ON THE DIRECTIONS

All words we utter,
all sound that comes through us is sacred.
We are channels through which creation occurs.
Each word we utter, each sound that moves through us
becomes all that we see, becomes the divine form.

Please stand up.

Face north. How far is north? Where is north? How close?
Face east. How far is east? Where is east? How close?
Face south. How far is south? Where is south? How close?
Face west. How far is west? Where is west? How close is west?
Face north. Face south. Face east. Face west. (Repeat four times.)

Look up. Look down. Look up. Look down. Look up. Look down.
Look behind you. Look behind you. What do you see?
Look in front of you. Look in front of you. What do you see?
Do not think. Just look.
Look to the left. Look to the right.
Look to the left. Look to the right.
Look up. Look down. Look up. Look down. Look up. Look down.
Look up. Look down. Look up. Look down. Look up. Look down.
Look to the Self.

Where are you, O Self? When will I find you?
I have looked to the north, I have looked to the south.
I have looked behind me, I have looked in front of me.
I have looked up, I have looked down.

I have been all around.
Where are you, O Self? May I find you?
That which you do not see is the Self. Seek that.

Om Shanti.

THE POWER OF SACRIFICE

How does a person reach greatness? How is a home built? How is a friend befriended? How does a relationship endure? How are great monuments built? How are children born? How do I continue to exist for you? How do you continue to exist for me?

Upon one word is built the foundation which enables us to endure a relationship, to bring life into the world, to build a house or a monument. The word is *sacrifice.*

Without sacrifice, not even love is possible. Love is not a thing that is "out there." We try to say love is this or that, but the minute you say love is, it isn't. Love is *neti, neti*, --no, no, no thing. It is not a thing. Then what is it? This you must find out. You see I can't say everything. The power of the *Guru* is to pull everything out of you.

There is a place called Sagara. There is a place called Jerusalem. There is a place called Mecca, a place called Medina. There is this place where we are. These places where people are seeking higher knowledge and where knowledge is imparted are holy ground, are places of sacrifice. In these places, the wise sacrifice. In Mecca and Medina, there is a great deal of power. Why? Because a life stood up to impart knowledge and to make the ignorant wise. In Jerusalem a life also was sacrificed. Sagara is the name of the place where Kapila spent his last days.

Do you know who Kapila was? He created the Sāṃkhya system. Kapila spent his last days on the banks of a river in Calcutta, the place of my birth. There he also sacrificed. Wherever you stand up and sacrifice, you make that place holy.

That place of sacrifice is full of pain and torture. Believe me, I know. Think of carrying a baby in the womb for nine months. It takes sacrifice to rear the child up, minute by minute, hour by hour, day by day. All of you who are mothers know what I am talking about. It takes a lot of sacrifice, and the sacrifice doesn't stop. Sacrifice does not stop.

Sacrifice is like the breath. You have to keep on breathing, or else what happens? You die! It takes sacrifice. You have to keep breathing. Sacrifice is like that. You can say, "I have a sore throat, I've got a headache, I have a fever, " but you still go on. You still go on breathing. Even though you say, "My chest hurts, my this hurts, my that hurts," you've got to keep on breathing. Sacrifice is like that. You have to keep on doing even though you are suffering. Sacrifice is suffering.

There are many thankless hearts in the world. You rarely get a "thank you" with a full heart. You wait for that golden day when that thank you will come after all your struggle, but no, you don't get it. You get crucified. Accept the cross. Like Christ said, "Take up your cross and follow me." Get nailed to the cross. Are you ready to do that? That's what spiritual life means. You have to keep on breathing and keep on sacrificing. You cannot wait for that thank you and hope that it will come.

Sacrifice is very, very powerful. At the same time it is a must, it is a necessity. It is a real need in life. It is needed. You yourself have to sacrifice every day. Sometimes you go to work when you have a bad fever. You could call in sick, but if you do that too much, you will be fired. So you have to sacrifice the pain. You endure that pain and go to work because you have to live. You sacrifice even for yourself. You keep on breathing. Breathing and sacrifice go hand in hand. Breath carries sacrifice and sacrifice carries breath.

Great monuments have never been built through fantasy and empty talk. "Oh, I'm going to do this and I'm going to do that." A monument is created through sacrifice. Sacrifice includes love, endurance, and devotion. It includes commitment and meditation. In sacrifice everything is included. Nothing escapes sacrifice.

When you find yourself not remembering the word sacrifice, it is because you have not embodied it yet. You have to embody it. It has to become your flesh. Then you will be able to get crucified. And you will love it. Then you will say, "Father, forgive them for they know not what they do."You will be able to let go even at that moment. Are you hearing what I am saying? Even at that moment you will forgive. You will even enjoy this crucifixion. The cup is bitter but the taste is sweet because there is nonpossession, there is the bliss of freedom. Sacrifice.

When you have a problem, remember your breath. You have to go through life inhaling and exhaling. Do not get stuck any place. The breath never gets stuck. It stops a moment, but it keeps going. It lets go. It goes into the inhalation, stops a moment, then goes into the exhalation. It goes into the exhalation, stops a moment, then goes back into the inhalation. That experience is going into *sat-chit-ānanda* (existence, knowledge and bliss), going into the fire of *Brahman* (the absolute). For a moment or two it all stops there. And then it goes on, continues. The breath keeps living.

We are conditioned to possess, to hold, to have the need for this and that. We tend to hold, to hold onto promises, to hold onto everything. But the great fact of life is that everything is subject to change. That is terrifying, isn't it? Every single thing is subject to change at any given moment. So why hold on? Just let it go. Let it go, but with sacrifice. How do you do that? You have to become a Yogi, you have to give birth to a Yogi. You have to become a *bodhisattva* (one whose essence is perfect knowledge). You have to take that golden oath of a *bodhisattva* which is to continue to meditate and sacrifice until all sentient beings are self-realized. That is how you live: survive, care for the other. Bring joy and laughter to another. Bring someone peace. Show someone the path. This must be lived.

With the mind we hold on and we don't want to sacrifice. But sacrifice occurs, regardless of how much we hold on. The way of life is like the breath. Inhale and exhale. Everything is subject to change and everything is moving. A child cries all night. A husband yells and screams. A wife is disappointed. There are so many suffering people in the world, and yet they survive. They cry one minute, and the next minute they are smiling. Everything is subject to change; nothing ever remains the same.

In our hearts we have to cultivate compassion. It is very hard to cultivate compassion in a land of plenty. If you want something, you go get it. There is no one to stop you. Sure, go and take whatever you want. You can have it, you can have it, sure, you can have it! One thing that is different between the East and the West is that in the East you find beggars everywhere. Everywhere you turn, there is a beggar looking for a handout, crying out, "Ma, Ma," constantly asking for something, constantly asking. And you are constantly giving.

In the East, it is very easy to cultivate compassion. The suffering is thrust right in your face. You see a leper in front of you, or a maimed person, or a mother with five kids. She is dragging five kids. Each child is holding onto the other, and they are pulling themselves through the street. Their bodies are all weak, and they are sick, almost dying out there on the road. But the mother is holding onto the five little ones and she is going. That is a woman for you. In America you do not see that. Over here, if you have no money you go to welfare. It is very nice, but everything is sanitized, you see, sanitized. You don't see the pain. In the East you can see the pain. It is very open. They come and pull out of you your compassionate heart. They pull it out of you and you cannot help but give. But you cannot give to all of them or you would die yourself.

Over here you do not have that opportunity to see the sick, the suffering, the maimed, the lunatics. What you see are mannequins, those meticulous looking things in the department stores with their nice clothes and plastic faces. You look at those nicely manicured and clean-cut things, and you think you are supposed to be like that. So what do you do? The average person becomes a mannequin too. What you see, you become.

So how are great places born? How is a home sustained? Through sacrificing, not by acquiring more things, not by having more new furniture, new curtains, new carpets. No, a lot of people think that they want to have a"nice" home. They do not want to have a home; they want to have a "nice" home. There is a difference between a nice home and a home. There is a difference. A home has warmth that comes from within. A home has care, care and warmth, not just gas and electric. A home secures and holds a relationship. It sustains through sacrifice.

To sacrifice you have to see the *other*. You have to see the other without demanding anything of the other. It is very hard to get anything from anyone. Everyone is needing and everyone is wanting. So how can you want from someone who is wanting and needing? Such people cannot give. As long as people are wanting or needing, they are in no position to give. They can be there as a body in your presence to reflect to you that you are also in that position. This is life, this is the truth, this is reality.

You have to see the other. To be a friend, you have to see someone and say, "Ah my friend, bewitched am I, caught in the rapture of one passing by. As the spinning goes on and the turning is there, I am caught in the rapture of one passing by." This is life, this is reality. We have to be there for the other. You have to be there with that feeling, with that heartfelt feeling of "This human being is not going to be here forever."

We depend on the security from the past. We think yesterday's situation will be the same today and will continue tomorrow. This is foolishness. This is real insecurity. We depend on *saṃskāras* (past impressions, incarnate structures); we depend on past impressions. Because he was there, or she was there, or they were there yesterday, we think they are going to be there tomorrow. Forget it! The Yogi lives just with today. There is no tomorrow. There is no yesterday, no past. Forget it! It is over! You must be in the moment without expecting anything from the other.

The only one you can expect something from is yourself. Expect how you can be warm in the moment. Give more and you will be amazed. You are like the ocean. You never dry up. You are full of wealth and power. You have everything. Feel you are the ocean, and in that moment be ready to give of yourself. But do not become vulnerable to the other's greed. Be watchful of it, mindful. Use your intelligence, because there are individuals who will exploit you. Beware of wolves in sheeps' clothing.

The power lies in the hands of the giver. The power also lies in the hands of the taker. Your damnation or your survival is in your hands, in your taking and in your giving. There is so much to life. Just live it one day at a time.

There are so many great lives that have lived. How did they become so great? Today we can sit and talk about their lives. Christmas is coming, and throughout the Christian world, people will be singing about Christ. Likewise, every year in the place called Sagara, all the devotees and all the people who do Yoga take pilgrimage to Sagara to remember Kapila and how he spent his last days in the cold and in the rain of the monsoons. He shrivelled up and left the body. But he gave to the world jewels that money cannot buy: knowledge, knowledge.

To live and coexist is very easy to do. It is very easy to live, me for you, and you for me. It seems easy to be for each other. But the *kleśās* (afflictions, hindrances) will not allow you to see it. The power of lust, the power of greed, the power of fear, the power of ignorance keeps us from knowing the reality and will not allow us to coexist peacefully.

Despite it all, we are very peaceful beings. We can exist peacefully, right? Don't you feel you can exist very peacefully? You can live and give to one another. Don't you feel you can do that? But why is it that we don't do it? The ego gets in the way. The play of illusion comes and does not allow the good to happen. This comes from the *kleśās*, from ignorance (*avidyā*), not knowing the reality of life, not knowing the truth. That reality can come only from embodiment. For that, one must sacrifice. Sacrifice is a must. There is no way out.

Om Shanti.

*MEDITATION EXERCISE: FACE TO FACE**

**Note: The following exercise as well as the others that follow are done during the meditations under the guidance of the Guru. They are meditation exercises and therefore reading them does them little justice; their power to transform comes about by* doing *them. Nevertheless, it is hoped that their inclusion here hints at their profundity and provides a sense of their power.*

Please stand up and walk.

In the going I am coming.
In the coming I am going.
I am coming. I am going.

Stand. Face each other.
We stand face to face.
Neither I see me, nor you see you.
Om Shanti.

Walk. (Several seconds elapse.)

Stand. Face each other.
We stand face to face.
Neither I see me, nor you see you.
Then, what is?
Om Shanti.

Continue to walk. (Several seconds elapse.)

Stand. Face each other.
We stand face to face.
Neither I see me, nor you see you.
Here I am and here you are.
Neither I see me, nor you see you.
What can you do for me?

What can I do for you?
We stand face to face
And neither I see me, nor you see you.
What can you do for me?
What can I do for you?
We stand face to face,
and neither I see me nor you see you.
Om Shanti.

Walk faster now...slow down.
Close your eyes. Continue to walk.
Open your eyes. Walk fast.
Stop and close your eyes.
Om Shanti.

Open your eyes and continue to walk.
Walk fast...now slow down.
Stop and face the other.
I am here, I am here so you can see.
I am here so you can see
the me that I do not know,
the me that I cannot see.
Om Shanti.

Continue to walk....
Stop and face each other.
We stand face to face.
Neither I see me, nor you see you.
Then where are we?
Where am I? Who am I, that you should
stop and look at me?
Om Shanti.

Continue to walk....
Stop.
Face north.
Face east.
Face west.
Face south.
(This is repeated five times.)
Look up. Look down. Look up. Look down.
Look up. Look down. Look behind you.
Look in front of you. Look up. Look down.
Look to the left. Look to the right.
Look in back of you. Look in front of you.
Look up. Look down. Look up. Look down.
Look behind you. Look in front of you.
Look up. Look down. Look up. Look down.
Look to the Self.

Om Shanti, Shanti, Shanti.

SUFFERING, FREEDOM AND APARIGRAHA

It takes a long time to become pure. It takes a long, long time. But we have to go through the fire of circumstance, of suffering. We have to feel it. We have to know how it burns us. And we will also come to the realization through the suffering and the burning that a thing in itself does not exist. So when you are suffering, don't think you are suffering by yourself. The whole world is suffering with you, especially those who are close to you, like your friends, your children, your relatives, your mother, your father. Everyone is suffering.

And then, when you are free, oh! That is a great day. That's a great day for merriment and giving thanks, because then everyone becomes free. Everyone feels the lightening of the burden, the pain, the suffering. Ah! So great! It's like being in a hospital and then being released. When a young patient comes in sick, the parents come in with the suffering child. Then follow the doctors and nurses, and all those tubes and injections. Everyone is saying "Oh, poor thing. I hope she gets well." And everybody is crying and has their fingers crossed. Finally, the patient is cured, the bills are paid, and everyone is happy.

It could be, though, that the patient doesn't learn from that suffering and the people around them don't learn. The suffering comes back and with that there is more pain. It comes back twice as bad. And so we have to go through the fire, the fire of suffering, the struggle. But it doesn't last forever. It gives everybody a jolt.

You have to go through the fire too. You have to eventually come to grips with yourself and really embody the meaning of *aparigraha*: nonpossessiveness, nonattachment, detachment. You come alone into this world and alone you leave it. You cannot take anyone with you. Furthermore, you cannot really depend on anyone. The only things to depend upon are knowledge and wisdom, because they will see you through. You cannot depend on another human being because everyone and everything is subject to change. At any given time he or she can get up and walk away.

Eventually, through the fire of suffering, the true meaning of *aparigraha* comes, and you begin to see that you have to learn to make friends with yourself. You have to see yourself and accept it. This I am. This I am. Fragile! This I am, caught in the midst of circumstances. This I am. This I am, coming from nowhere into this place where I am, nowhere. This I am.

We have to come to grips with that. Through it, we come to see how important *aparigraha* is. And when we begin to see that, we begin to truly give. Give. Not just giving so that we can get back a compliment, but giving for the sake of purification, to empty ourselves. To empty all the things that we have around us. You keep on giving, giving, until you have given everything and you feel exhausted from the giving of things. Then comes the next stage of giving. You give up aggressiveness, you give up aversion, you give up hate, you give up anger, you give up possessiveness. You give up believing "I have to have it my way, or else." This giving up is of a different nature. It is a gradual movement.

Giving up anger is a very hard thing to do. A lot of people are very angry. I hope you are not like that. Are you angry? Who's angry? "I'm angry at the world. They all did me in. They all did me wrong. My mother let me down, my father let me down, my sister. He won't do this, she won't do that. Me, me. I, I am angry. I'm angry at the world." You have to give up that anger, you see, after the giving of *things* has been exhausted. With this, a certain emotional stickiness also comes to an end. Then what do you have? Then you have love. Pure love, which says, "I love you, no matter who you are."

You have to give up those icky, sticky, gummy states that you exist through, that keep your world of neuroses alive. Once all that is done, you have nothing but love. And you say: "So what! I'll walk another mile! I'll give another hug! I'll give another plate of food!" After the sticky, gummy affairs are over, you can say that you see. But then, you see even more. You see that it is very hard, because the tentacles of your ego are stuck in the gum of circumstance. You know you're stuck in it. You cannot get out of it. Your tentacles are stuck in it, your senses are stuck. Those sticky conditions in us won't let us live, won't let us just be in the moment or let us say, "I love you" and truly mean it. Hence, we need *aparigraha*. It was with good reason that Patañjali (author of the *Yoga Sūtrās*) taught *aparigraha*. It is a very beautiful discipline.

There is another part of this sticky, gummy affair that causes one to say, "Why should I care anymore? Everything is subject to change, so why should I bother? I'll just give up." So you get into a worse state. It's like "Crazy Glue!" That's a real hard mess to come out from. Just because the flower is going to change doesn't mean that I'm not going to enjoy its beauty while it is. See how pretty they are, these flowers on the *havan* (altar). Just because they are going to decay and die does not mean that I'm not going to worship and honor them while they last, and look upon them with affection. This we must do. They are subject to change, and they will go. But they will be transformed. The mind that is not yet alive and aware does not see the stages of transformation. We see flowers wither and die and the petals fall off. We throw them away. But during the process, many of us are not seeing. We don't care about what's happening, so we do not see. Yet the transformation is taking place. The power of life continues. Nothing is wasted.

The culmination of all these stages and transformations is existence, knowledge, and bliss. Cultivate thoughts like, "This I did not know. This I will find out. Therefore, I will do my *sādhana* (Yoga practice)." To know it with the mind and to hear it from the wise that you are existence, knowledge and bliss is not sufficient. You must experience this truth as embodiment.

Om Shanti.

THE MYTH OF INDEPENDENCE, THE TRUTH OF INTERDEPENDENCE

Today people are very confused. When we consider previous generations and compare them to the present one, we see such a contrast, such a difference. The difference, however, is only in lifestyle. The essential underlying unity of all human existence is the need to be. This requires that one cooperate so that one may survive through the other. This interdependence underlies all human existence.

The calling of today's society is to be independent. This is such a hard thing to accomplish. To be independent means to stand alone. According to the wise this is not possible. This cannot be. So, one ought to practice another way. Instead of striving for independent living, one has to learn the art of interdependence. Interdependence. This calls attention to the importance of the *other* in our lives. Interdependence. This means waiting on the other for our survival. But the call in today's society is, "I know everything, I am independent." Because of this, the poor and innocent suffer so much. Four or five generations ago, the elders were very much respected. Today there are no elders. The youth of today are saying, "I'm an adult! I'm independent! Treat me like an adult!" And they look at their parents-- who are truly adults-- and they say this, not for a moment realizing they are facing true adults. Because of this, young people are suffering very badly. The elders are suffering also because they are baffled and do not know what to do.

This is part of a new movement going on. A universal change is occurring. All of us had better wake up to this reality. All of you sitting here left home years ago. "I'm seventeen, I'm eighteen. I've got to go now, I've got to do it on my own. I have to do my thing. I have to do rock music. I have to dance. I have to shake, I have to show the world I'm here. Look at me, look at me!" All of you walked out; some of you were told to leave, were told, "Get out of here!" But you left, nevertheless!

In today's life one has to learn the art, the science and the philosophy of interdependence. I need you and you need me. Give to me and I will give to you. Together we can be. This is the art of interdependence. Forget about independence. It is a fantasy. You always need someone. You need a boss to pay you. You need a car to drive. You need the government because this is an ordered society. You need these things.

You need your family to support you when you are down and out, when no one cares about you. If your friends have left you, you need your family. It's survival. You cannot say then, "I'm an adult!" What does that mean? The notion of independence is a cultural fantasy. Hence, the art of interdependence must be cultivated. "I need you, my sister, so I can talk to you about my deeply felt emotions. I need you, my brother, because you are a man in my presence, and you were born from the same womb. I need you." Let your brother know you need him and let your sister know you need her. You have to let your mother know you need her. You have to let your father know you need him.

The art of interdependence is a science, it is a philosophy. It is something that is much neglected. There is a lot of suffering in the world. We live here in our own little cubicles and think everything's running fine. Life is cozy. But look closer. There is mass confusion all over the world, not just here. Suffering is everywhere.

Women had better wake up. They have heard from their great-grandparents and especially their grandmothers and mothers how hard it is to be a woman. They hear again and again how hard it is to take care of the kids all the time. So now, the modern woman says, "I'm not going to do what my great-grandmother did: stay home and just crochet and knit!" Women have become very angry.

But remember the grandmothers of years gone by. It was so nice to cuddle up next to your grandmother. She always made you feel so secure. My granddaughter still comes to cuddle up with me, because she knows that I'm not going to say, "You're too heavy! Get out of here!" She knows that no matter how much she jumps and pulls at me it doesn't hurt. She is not here for me; she is the one who needs help to survive. I am here for her.

You have to act because through your actions the worlds live. The worlds are born out of our actions. What we do is important, more so than what we think. This interdependence is so important, and so neglected.

Interdependence is very vital. The little plant you might have sitting in your room needs water to survive. So you water it. From time to time, you have to turn it around to face the sun. During those times, you are giving that plant its existence. But at the same time you need that plant for its beauty, its presence. It is giving you a perspective through which you will come alive. It is breathing like you and like me. Interdependence. Everything has that nature. Without the *other*, there is no you.

Om Shanti.

THE PROBLEM OF NEGATIVITY... BRINGING IN THE POSITIVE!

A great deal of anger must be eliminated to see the significance of interdependence. If you are angry where can you go and what can you do? You get more angry. And if you hate? What happens to that anger or that hate? It turns on you. The result is chronic illness, an inability to cope with circumstances. Inability to cope is a result of hate. So you have to forgive. You might not forget, but you can forgive. In order to forgive, the third *sūtra* of the second pada of Patañjali's *Yoga Sūtra* must be realized. This sūtra describes the five *kleśas* (afflictions, hindrances), the impurities of ignorance, egoism, attachment, aversion and clinging to life-- *avidyā, asmitā, rāga, dveṣa, abhiniveśa.* Hatred stems from these five *kleśas.*

When you hate, whose responsibility is it? It's yours of course. You're the one who has the hate. Your hate is an inability to cope. You hate not because someone is doing you wrong. You actually hate yourself for not being able to manage your own affairs. You hate because you cannot cope. Of course, you'll lash out at this one and scream at that one, yell at this one and walk out on that one. You might stay out all night, or even get drunk or open yourself up to abuse. Many people do this just to fight back. But this is horrendous, this is stupid.

And in the end, what do you have? A tired body, a weak nervous system. The mind is in a fog. Hence, the importance of interdependence must be stressed upon everyone. Our need for one another is the rule of life. Life always includes the other, there is no way out of it. It is life's law.

Why do you think we are confronted with the opposite? We are always facing something. Why? Because we have to move it out of the way. The only way we can move the other out of the way so that we can be free is to pay the price. Every time someone comes and stands in front of you with a negative appearance or attitude, he is telling you or she is telling you, "Come on, you owe me a debt! Come on, you are going to have to pay it today!" But we are unable to cope with the other. The art of interdependence is not practiced, so we get affected by the negative influences, we become tense. We walk away or become silent, or we creep out of the room. But we cannot run away. That *other* is going to be around again and again until the debt is paid. The debt has to be erased.

The negative and the positive. If something positive appears you welcome it. This is a karmically formed affair. But there is also the negative karmic affair, past impressions and expressions coming back in a negative way because you didn't work them out. The negative comes back.

Sometimes the negative comes back as a mood. You know how rotten these moods are. They are like glue. The mood clings to you, gets stuck to you because you have that negativity too. You get affected , and you have to pay the price.

Don't run away from negativity. Confront it, confront it! By first confronting it in yourself before you speak a word to the other person, you accept the situation. "Yes, I am feeling emotionally disturbed right now because of the appearance of this person in my life. I can't stand this person. I wish he or she would go to Timbuktu." This shows you have a debt to pay, just like the money lenders who come and say, "Come on, pay up." These feelings will come over and over again until the affair is resolved. The slate must be wiped clean.

You know you have to pay your debt. You have to pay up. Compared to this kind of debt a credit card is nothing. But you have to resolve these negativities. Confront them! Stand up to them, not to fight, but to discriminate them away.

For this to take place, what should we do? There is a beautiful *sūtra* that provides a solution: when a negative thought comes you have to replace it with a positive one. Say to yourself in Sanskrit, "*pratipakṣa-bhāvanam*," the cultivation of the opposite. When a negative influence comes into your life and you feel the emotional stress of it, you have to replace it with a positive influence. Smile and say, "Hello, how are you? Would you like a cup of tea? I know you are angry with me, but right now I would like to have a cup of tea. Would you like to have a cup of tea with me?" It takes a little doing, but you have to pay your debt. You've got to pay up the debt and no amount of money is going to do it.

The negativity is embodied in the nervous system, and it has to be gotten out. So you practice *pratipakṣa-bhāvanam*, the cultivation of the opposite. Try that for a change. Through it you develop the art of true living, and you realize the need for interdependence. "I need you." Don't be afraid to say that. "I need you." Don't be proud. Pride comes from the *kleśas*: *avidyā, asmitā, rāga, dveṣa, abhiniveśa*. It is very easy to say, "I need you, let's stop playing all those games, I need you." It's very easy to do anything after that.

What do you *really* need? Usually people say they need money. Does a piece of paper solve your problem? No, it doesn't. Once you get money, you cannot keep it. It goes away. Once you realize this, you won't have any use for money anymore, at least not in your old way. You will see it's so great to have another life in front of you, a warm vibrant being in front of you. This is better than a piece of paper, much better.

It is up to us to create a positive circumstance at all times. Therefore, we always have to use our intelligence and be on our toes. You have to be like a sword fencer. You have to be quick, be able to take out your sword of intelligence and say, "On guard, I'm here!" You have to be ready all the time; you cannot take time off from life. Always try to bring in the positive.

Sometimes in the fire of circumstance there is a slip of the tongue. You may say something negative instead of positive. In that case you must forgive yourself and say, "A slip of the tongue is no fault of the mind." If anyone complains, explain that it was just a slip of the tongue and you didn't really mean to say it. This does happen.

We're always involved in circumstance and situation. Always give someone something that will raise his or her awareness. Don't discourage people with anything that will pull them down. Don't even give them a dollar if you think they will abuse it. Don't do that. Don't give them anything if it's going to bring them down, even though you may be dying to give it to them. Just say, "No, I love you too much."

If someone asks for a dollar to buy cigarettes, distract him or her. I have all kinds of cloves and little chewables I carry in my purse, little spices of all kinds. If someone wants a smoke, I say, "Here, try one of these." Before long, the person says, "I don't need a cigarette." It takes a while, but the need eventually disappears. Try not to encourage the weakness of another.

Human beings have both strength and weakness. If you keep encouraging the weakness, it begins to get fat. Yes, fat! Then it takes anything it can get its hands on, with no concern for the consequences. But if you bring out the strength, you can see how great a human being can become. Very, very great.

You have power and weakness. You have courage and fear. They are always battling to see which one gets the upper hand, which one is going to be the winner. There's always a game. "Let's see which one is going to win out today, my weakness or my strength." Encourage your strength, overcome your weakness and fear.

Om Shanti.

HAPPINESS AND PERFECTION

Bring happiness into the world. Every single day we should strive to make somebody happy. Not to make yourself happy, but to make someone else happy. Go out of your way to make someone happy today. Let that be a rule of life. If you have no one to make happy but you do have a cat, buy it some catnip today. Every day make someone happy. Start with those closest and move out from there. Make someone happy each and every day.

It is a beautiful rule to make people happy, to see the smiles on their faces, to see their eyes bright with joy. It's a great thing to see, especially when you do this for someone you do not like. What great elation you feel! To make someone you like happy is easy. But find someone who you don't like or who you are having problems with and make *that one* happy. It's a great challenge to do that! Find a way, and I'm sure you'll locate a ticklish spot somewhere in that person. Then the laughter starts, a change takes place. It takes a little doing, but it can be done.

When you make that human being who you didn't like turn around and like you, then you're on top of the world. You can have anything, you can do anything. Try to make the one you have despised happy, the one you haven't liked and the one who doesn't like you. If you do this, soon you will be hunting in this world for everyone you cannot stand. I'm doing it. I can see a lot of ugliness in a lot of people, but I'd rather not let it make me feel bad. So what I do is try to look at a person's positive side. Everybody has a positive side. Start with that. It may be their smile or walk. Find something you can like about that distasteful person. Like it and it will grow.

There is more to like than not to like because we are existence, knowledge, and bliss. Even that distasteful person is existence, knowledge, and bliss. All this is *Brahman*, the absolute. All this is from the absolute. Everything is consciousness. Therefore, nothing is imperfect. The imperfection lies only in our thinking.

As we think, so we act. In actuality, there are no imperfections. The imperfections that we see are opportunities to manifest the great perfection at the heart of life. The imperfections give us a purpose to create perfection. When you see an imperfect situation, know that you have a job lined up for you to do, something to make perfect and something to make *you* perfect. The messy bed gives you a purpose. The dirty dish gives you a purpose. The person filled with sorrow and confusion gives you a purpose. Once you fulfill your purpose, you say, "Oh, how great!" A satisfaction is felt.

Aim for that satisfaction every day in people, in circumstances. There are plenty of perfect messes around for us to perfect. Try to clean them up. If someone's life is too hard, give that person a hand, help clean it up. If someone's car is not working, help fix it. Bring laughter into that person's life. Bring joy, give a little bit of your life to another. It is needed.

Om Shanti.

MEDITATION EXERCISE- STANDING AND SITTING

Please stand up.

Look at your feet.
Now sit down, very slowly.
Very slowly get up again.
Watch your feet.
This is a meditation in motion.
Very slowly sit down again.
Watch your feet.
(This is repeated three times.)

Feel the motion.
Feel how every limb of your body is moving.
Feel the total body contact.
(The standing and sitting movement
is repeated three more times.)

It is by doing this type of meditation
over and over again
that one begins
to acknowledge the reality of life.
(The motion is repeated three more times.)

Experience your whole body move.
This is meditation in motion.
(Three more repetitions.)

You can never see under your feet.
Even if you lift up your feet and try to look under them,
it does not work.
Why can you never see under your feet?
There is a reason for that.
It is like the top of your head.
You can never see the top of your head.
You can never see your back.

Although you may look at another's back
or you may look in a mirror,
your back is forever hidden from you.
You can never see your eyes.

Om Shanti, Shanti, Shanti.

PAIN AND THE LESSON OF BEING

There are many paths in life. The eyes are always looking everywhere. Look and you find that wherever we look, the pleasure comes with the pain, and together with the pain comes the release. The pain is a very beautiful ecstasy. It takes you to the core of your existence, more so than pleasure does. Pleasure tells you how nice it could be. But pain tells you that you must be.

Pain is a real friend, a true friend. Do not look at pleasure and pain as something ugly or disgusting or as a problem in life. Pleasure and pain appear to be a problem because we do not feel. A real friend brings you real gifts. Pain is a wonderful friend; it makes you feel. This is its gift. You don't believe me, do you? Strange though it may seem, it is true! Pain is a beautiful friend. Pain makes you cry. Pain makes you say, "I'm hurting." Pain makes you say "I'm sorry." Pain makes you say, "I'm suffering, that's enough!" Pain helps you say, "I give up, I surrender." All of these are beautiful experiences. If you could write down all the benefits of pain, you would say, "Give me more, give me more." You learn so much from pain.

Through pain you learn to have a positive rather than a negative attitude. Pain helps you to discover the smile on the other's face. Pain helps you provide for yourself and for others. Pain helps you to remember that pain will come again and again and again, until you can be in that place of perfect surrender.

One has to cry. Many people cannot cry because they have cried so much and they have been hurt so much that they have developed an indifference. They say, "So what?" The tears are used up and there is a parched feeling inside. They have not yet realized that pain is like a stick of dynamite; it clears things away. After a person has lived with pain for some time, he or she becomes like sparkling gold. One begins to shine like gold after that pain. After pain has purified you, you do not have to learn how to surrender or how to cry. You can just be. It becomes a way of life. You will always be surrendered and you will live through your heart. The heart has to change. It is necessary to cry, and the pain helps you to cry.

You must watch your attitudes. There are too many people locked into a negative attitude. Be in the spirit, be in *samādhi* (absorption). Be in the now. Be, be !

Om Shanti.

THE EYE OF WISDOM

You must look with the eye of wisdom, not with the eye of ignorance. Look with the eye of wisdom. How may one cultivate this way of seeing? The eye of wisdom is cultivated through understanding. Understanding comes through listening and reading. When you find a book that has words of wisdom in it, pick it up gently and respect it wholeheartedly. Learn to change life. Change not only your own life, but everyone's. Wherever you go, clear the pathway as you walk. Everywhere you go, as you look around, make things clean. This does not merely mean cleaning up your own mess. It means cleaning up the people around you too. As you walk in front of someone, be a mirror for them. But you have to be clean if they are to see themselves in you.

Om Shanti.

MEDITATION EXERCISE: PERSPECTIVES

Sit up straight please.
Now look to the side.
Now look behind you. Now look in front of you.
What did you see?

Now look again. Now look to the right.
Now look forward.
Did the scenery change for you, from this side to that side to here? Did it change?

Did you see the difference?
Looking at this side there is a particular view, looking at that side another view, looking in front, another view. Look, look again.
Look with the intentness to see.

It might be your last time looking at this.
So look, live in such a way that every moment could be your last.

Om Shanti.

THE YOGA OF ACTION (KARMA YOGA)

In every action there is a reaction in thought, word and deed. If you watch very closely you will experience the intimacy between cause and effect, the law of life. When one is educated through the guidance of dedicated teachers, sacred writing, concentration, meditation, and internal and external purifications, thought becomes concentrated on one's object of desire. Then one begins to understand cause and effect.

When one knows, action is appreciated. There is joy in one's realizing that action produces creation. Every movement is a movement of infinity. It is in action that we can go on and on and on. The realization of the infinite comes with accepting the world of action. They cannot be kept apart.

This world is a manifestation of the unmanifest. In this world there is vibration, activity, creation, sound, form and color, which all play prominent roles in our lives. We cannot stop looking. We sustain this existence through our existence. In the looking, hearing, smelling, tasting and touching there is action. Because we enjoy these sensations, we create possibilities wherein and whereby we produce more of the same, and in bountiful proportions.

Men, women and children are always reaching out of the bondage of obscurity, sometimes thoughtfully as adults, or playfully as children. The need to be free is to escape from not being known to being known. Men, women and children can never be content with just the bare necessities of life: food, shelter and clothing. So we occupy ourselves with other things. For example, we build societies, structures and superstructures that express our need to be free. Yet in the building and in the need to be free, there is the fear of destruction. We cannot bear the thought of this. Therefore, we go on through pain and pleasure, laboring through many trying circumstances because we must transcend what is, in order to become what we are yet to be. In this there is pleasure; in this there is pain.

Individuals must carry out their principles of life according to their understanding. In so doing, we go through life constantly expanding and penetrating in order to become. Sometimes in the maze of life, we become confused and lost. We lose sight of our intentions; we become afraid. However, these interruptions cannot stop us. We have to keep moving.

Our life is manifested through our actions. We live in two worlds: the inner and the outer. These worlds are interdependent. We act in the outer world and in doing so make the inner world known.

We want to live a total, wholesome life, and we can only do so if we consider the whole. To do this we have to go to the great philosophies of the past and acquire the understanding therein. Then, upon introspection, we will appreciate the outer and the inner, the manifest and the unmanifest. A joy will fill our hearts. There will be, through this understanding, a reason and a need for performing actions in the world.

The urgency of doing and becoming allows us to constantly remain on the move. This movement is wonderful only if there is joy in the completed action. Life is a flux of three moments: past, present and future. We have to balance our lives with strength and understanding; cause and effect must be respected. All our actions and reactions must be dedicated to Self-realization, which is the reason for our being. The individual and universal must be in close contact all the time. Never must the mind stray from this unity, for it is in this joy that there is ecstasy.

Unity is a beautiful thought; harmony is welcomed by all. Where can we find it? Many have yearned for this knowledge, and many have failed in the pursuit of this wisdom. This knoweldge does not come by sheer wishing. However, indirect understanding is not difficult to acquire. There are thousands of books, radio and television programs on the subject. Anyone you meet is ready to give you information, opinions, and sometimes, against your wishes, they will try to help you. But there is nothing in this whole world that will convince you of the truth other than the experience of direct perception. It changes your whole life.

Fear is easily overcome by the Yoga of action, selfless action. Work on, just to keep the wheel of life moving. Give thanks and praises for the bounty of life.

When the *buddhi* (intellect) reasons, *viveka* (discrimination) is attached to the Yoga of action. Then the result is freedom, and in freedom nothing is ever stagnant. Consider the river flowing into the ocean. Watch how the day slips into the night. See the rainfall disappearing into the earth. Go into a vegetable garden which produces food for all. Walk by a flower garden. The fragrance is inhaled by all: the good, the bad, the indifferent. The same is true of the sun, spreading its rays upon all. Watch also how childhood gives way to youth, and youth gives way to maturity. The fullness of life is in the giving: giving birth, giving alms, being responsible in sustaining the continuation of birth and rebirth.

Again I must emphasize that *buddhi* is important for true Yoga of action to be accomplished. Selfless action requires more than merely abandoning the fruits of action. Selfless action requires reason and *viveka*. One must discriminate the real from the unreal, the eternal from the temporal. Time and time again, the individual who does not discriminate falls into the trap of delusion when performing worldly actions. He finds himself still lingering in attachments which give rise to desire. When desire remains unrewarded, it gives way to anger, restlessness and confusion. When this condition sets in, the reasoning capacity is weakened. We see and experience destruction all around; a restless mind can never have peace.

Yoga is skill in karma (action). One is not advised to ignore worldly duties. One can perform excellent work through the Yoga of action and come to the realization of selflessness. As a snake sheds its skin, as a skin is removed from an onion, as soap and water cleanse the body, the impressions and attachments will slip away a little at a time as the Yoga of action becomes perfected. Then surrender becomes a real and pure undertaking.

Om Shanti

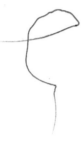

THE SILENT LANGUAGE

The spiritual path demands everything. Everything you have, not everything you *can* give but everything you *have* to give. There is no way out of it, absolutely no way. When one really feels the spiritual impact, the beauty and the thrill of being one hundred percent attached and one hundred percent detached is seen. It is a state of ecstasy. It also is the state at the core of our existence, but some know and some do not.

Everything around us is born of mind. We must strive through the mind for that perfection that Yoga teaches us: that Yoga is *citta-vṛtti-nirodhaḥ* (cessation of mental modifications). Come to understand this. Yoga is no mind, *citta-vṛtti-nirodhaḥ*. To go into that unmanifest state, you have to be like a little child. Christ said, "Suffer the little children to come unto me and forbid them not, for such is the kingdom of heaven." What did he mean by that? Little children have no mind. They are in the state of *citta-vṛtti-nirodhaḥ*. The children are nonpossessive, nonattached. They eat but they do not know what they eat; they just eat it if they like it. They take in everything in sight, drawing it into themselves. Yet, when you ask them what they ate, their answer is often silence. Mum is the word. They seem to say, "Ask me no questions, I'll tell you no lies." This is because they are mindless, they have no mind. And so Christ said, "Suffer the little children to come unto me and forbid them not, for such is the kingdom of heaven."

Adults have learned the power of language. With conditioned, cultural language we compromise and adulterate everything in sight. We play a game of words. Through our words we protect ourselves and manipulate the *other*. With the adult, anything goes. This creates stress and suffering. The adult is attached and possessive.

Children, on the other hand, do not have this problem. Because they have no mind, they cannot deliberately hurt anyone. They take anything and are satisfied with it for the moment. They are free to be and free to go. But, because they do not know exactly where they are going, they are pulled by the hand and taken here and taken there. The culture moves them, coming at them in the form of adults. However, the reverse can also be true. If the adult holds back and pays close attention to little children, that person is brought to *nirodhaḥ.* Children bring you to that state of no mind. Learn from children how to look at and yet not name things. Try it. Just look. Do not name. Just look and be. Do not possess. Do not give any value to things; just look. The essence of life is beyond time and beyond place, beyond attributed values, beyond.

In the world of culture, in the world of human relations, we have to name everything. In communities, we have to speak the language of that community. We have to say, "This is a cup, give me a glass of water." We have to use language. This is not so in spiritual life. In spiritual life, in the essence, in the moment, there is *nirodhaḥ*, there is that silence.

So then what does spiritual life mean in society, in community? Societies have certain fixed ideas about what a spiritual individual is and is not. It is said that a spiritual person has to be like this or be like that. Some societies say that a spiritual person has no feelings, or a spiritual person doesn't drink, doesn't drive, doesn't get sick. If you look at any group or society, it has fixed ideas about how people should behave. But any sort of prescribed "behaving" is something that is against our nature, our true nature. We really don't want to behave in a way that is prescribed. It goes against our nature, our true nature, because we are born free, we are born with *nirodhaḥ*. Anything that is put on us, any requirement to toe the line goes against our grain. We want to break out. We want to be free, we want to feel free.

The question is, where can this freedom be felt? You cannot be free in society. You have to be free in the Self. Free in the Self. How do you do it? When do you do it? What circumstance allows for it? Who will understand you? All this is unimportant when that state of *nirodhaḥ* is embodied. Unimportant, because in the state of *nirodhaḥ* you will automatically be in the *ṛta* (truth, norm, sacred order) and that will guide you no matter where you are. You will go into it and come out of it, but you will not be tainted at all.

It is hard work trying to live in society and live a spiritual life because you can never appease society. Society wants to claim you. But you cannot be claimed by anyone. You have to say, "I am in this world but I am not of this world. I am here, but I am not here." Who can see that? Who knows that? That, indeed, is a state of *nirodhaḥ*: to be in this world but not of it. Or you can change it around and say, "I am of this world but I am not in this world." Either way you are in the state of *nirodhaḥ*.

Separate yourself through language. Watch the words you say. Watch who is speaking to you. Realize the significance and the power of words. Words are very, very powerful. Words are sacred. Each word is a *mantra* (instrument of thought, speech, sacred text). Each word has purity, vibration, sensation, sound, Each word makes the body. Words are sacred, words are very powerful. When someone says something nice to you, you feel good. The body releases some tension inside and gives itself over to a state of equilibrium. But the minute something negative is said, the body roars, it tears itself apart, it rips you inside. This is the power of words. Words make the body, words make the world. They are makers of place and circumstance. Words are powerful, words are sacred.

Hence, Yoga is *citta-vṛtti-nirodhaḥ*, the stopping of all words. I love that place. It's a place that allows me to be in all places. That place, when it is known, allows you to be in any place at any time, one hundred percent attached, one hundred percent detached. You want to be a Mohammed, you want to be a great soul, you want to be a Christ, you want to be a Gautama Buddha. You want to have knowledge, wisdom, understanding. You want to be able to work wonders in the world. Why? Because you see there is so much suffering. That place has to be known, that place beyond all words. Without knowing it, without feeling it, without embodying it, without living in that place, nothing can be accomplished.

Om, Shanti.

THE POWER OF OM

In the early writings of Eastern philosophy, in the sacred books such as the *Vedas*, the *Upaniṣads* and the *Bhagavad Gītā*, the word *Om* is pronounced before any other word. It holds a very high place. *Om* is to be chanted when you feel sick or happy or sorrowful. When you are going to bed, when you wake up in the morning, that word must come out of your mouth.

The word *Om* is a conscious application of an internal realization. How is this so? Because sound is always in you. You are born of sound. You cannot say hello without opening your mouth. You are born of sound and you continue through sound.

Words are always pouring from my mouth, but until I open these lips no sound comes out. Without sound, you cannot say "me," you cannot say "you," you cannot say "water" or "flower" or any other word. You cannot utter another's name without sound.

Try opening your mouth and see what comes out. For instance, say the word "mother." Good, I hear you. Now, close your mouth and before you say the word audibly, feel in your mouth how it is being formed. See if you can find the sound and the utterance of *Om* locked in the word "mother." Now, say the word out loud. Try to find *Om* in it.

There are three points to *Om*: the letters A, U and M. *Aum* and *Om* are the same. Every word has three points to it: a beginning, a middle and an end. Open your mouth. That is the first point. You then have to let the word move out. That is the second point. Finally, you have to shut your mouth. That is the third point. Three points, three *guṇas* (three components of experience: light, activity and inertia) compose the *Om*. Every word you utter has the same three points: first, the opening of the mouth, second, the expression of the sound that it carries, and third, the closing of the mouth.

Om is very sacred. *Om* is in every letter of the alphabet. It is in every consonant; it is in every vowel. It is in every word, in everything. It is tied up, wrapped up in everything. It is there. Although you may not hear it, you cannot say it is not there. It is in any word you say. You have to open your mouth. You have to let it out through sound. And you have to close your mouth.

Om. It is so quick, it is like a lightning flash. It goes so fast. The sacred sound *Om* is so fast and so close to you. Every word, every letter, every language, everyone throughout the world, every living being has to utter that sacred sound. No matter what sound is made, no matter what is said, it has three junctures: the opening, the letting out, and the completion. It is beautiful. And when you know that, how can you hate anyone? You are everyone, and everyone is you. You become one in the spirit. There is no difference between "I love" and "I hate." There is no separation: there is no hate, there is no love. But there is a unity that is beyond the cultural fantasies of everyday living.

The word *Om* has the three *guṇās*. When you open your mouth, the past, the present and the future are locked in that word. The flux of three moments is but a moment for all eternity. Each word you say goes around and around and spins and spins and spins. Words create action; action maintains the being of language. Words are the expression of your situation. Every word you say either confirms or destroys the circumstances of society, of nation, of culture. So, when you speak to destroy something, you better know what you are doing, because in destroying it, you also destroy yourself. And in the creation you also create yourself. So whatever we do, whatever we say, however we act, we are the world. In that moment we are creating our life, or in that moment we are destroying it. As a result of this, some people are happy, some people are sad. Many people are laughing, many people are also crying.

There is not one word you can say that does not have *Om* in it, not one single word. You might respectfully say, "I'm going to chant *Om* now," prayerfully attending to that sacred time, offering up praises and acknowledgment to the sacred sound of *Om*. But *Om* is more than just prayerful chanting. *Om* is found in every letter of the alphabet, in every vowel, in every consonant. In every language, everyone is saying *Om* every day. When you hear a baby cry, there you hear *Om*. What a beautiful sound that baby makes when it cries. It is *Om*. When you hear a baby cry, it is not just crying. It is creating, it is destroying through the power of *Om* that is within all of us. It is using the power of sound, the power of language, the power of the word.

During the course of the day, every day of the week, find some time to just sit and chant *Om*. Find the time to do it. Create your own sound. Your own music will be born. You do not have to learn it from someone else. Just open your mouth and chant. Beautiful sounds will come out from another world, another dimension. Just ride with it, take it to the extent you can take it. Let beautiful sounds be heard.

Om Shanti.

MEDITATION EXERCISE: FACING THE OTHER

Stand up please.
Walk a little.
Now stop and face the other.
I am in this world
but not of this world.
I am of this world
but not in this world.

Experience this.
We are here, but we are not here.
Then where are we?
Om Shanti.

Continue walking.
Stand and face the other.
We are in this world
but we are not of this world.
Om Shanti.

Continue walking.
Stop and face the other.
Who are you and who am I?
Why do I have to stand in front of you?
The other, the other
is your greatest challenge in life,
your liberator, your witness.

Om Shanti.

NONDUALITY AND THE OTHER

The power of the *other* is so strong. Are you frightened of the other standing in front of you? Do you think to yourself, "What will you have me do for you? What do you want out of my life anyway?" We try to spend as little time as we can in front of the other. If you spend a great deal of time in front of the other you will become one with the other.

It may be asked, "What are we afraid of when faced with the other?" Nonduality! This is something that cannot be known with the conditioned mind. You are familiar with duality. It is a conditioned reality of the manifest world. But people do not talk about nonduality. They talk about social living, about circumstances. You all know about duality. But how can nonduality be known? It is nonpossessiveness. There is nothing there. How can you live in that? And yet everyone must learn to live in nonduality because that is the way things really are. We run away from that which is real. People are scared, petrified. You stand in front of someone and immediately you are afraid of the unity; the power of duality is clouding your mind. You are afraid of being judged. You are afraid of being told you are ugly. You are afraid of criticism from the other.

The challenge is to find nonduality in duality. To do this, you have to practice *aparigraha* (non-possession). Give something away every day. You will begin to see that you will be giving away your *saṃskārās* (past impressions, incarnate structures), your attachments, your possessiveness. You will even give away the desire to not give anything away. You will begin to forget, "This is mine, this is an heirloom, this is something I have had for ages. This is something that my grandmother gave me from my great, great grandmother. This thing is inherited; I have it and I do not want to part with it." These types of thoughts will begin to disappear. In the end you will have to give it all up. You have to die. So you may as well give a little away every day, consciously. It is a great thing to give things away consciously. Why be taken by surprise? Why leave everything with a feeling of still being attached?

The law of karma says with every cause there is an effect. With every effect there is a cause. For every reaction there is an action; for every action there is a reaction. You just keep going around and around. You cannot get off the wheel. But the Yogi gets off the wheel of life and watches the merry-go-round. You see, there is a time when you are stuck in the world and then there comes a time when, through conscious spiritual evolution, you get out of life while still in this body. You get off the wheel of life and you watch the world going around through the actions and reactions of day to day circumstances. You must learn to live this way. You have to see the whole picture. This is why nonduality is so important.

The *other* is that link that will either make you or break you. The other can release you from *saṃskāra* and *kleśās* (afflictions, hindrances), or the other will help you to reestablish and confirm your *kleśās*. The other will do that to you. So you have to see the other and know there is a purpose for the other to be there. The other is there for us to serve, not to take from. Serve the other. You have to serve. Do you know why? So that the negative impressions will not stay, so that negative impressions will not react in negative ways. You have to serve the other.

You can change the power of the *guṇas*. You can change the power of *saṃskārās* and *kleśās* through the process of serving someone else. By giving service you clear the path. You clear it. You are not taking, you are giving. In giving, you are practicing nonattachment and in nonattachment there is liberation. This is very easy if you remember it every single day. To do this, chant *Om* as often as you can, especially when you get frightened. Take a deep breath and say *"Om."* Then exhale out the negative feelings arising in your body. Become strong and exhale the negativity out, using the words *shanti, shanti*. *Shanti* is peace. Say *"Om Shanti "* when you go to sleep at night. You will have a peaceful, restful sleep, even if it is only for one hour. But you have to let yourself go into that sacred place, the sacred place which you are.

The *other* in our life is very important and brings to us many opportunities. Why was the world created in such a way that we always come face to face with the other? Why is life this way? We are not here, and yet we are here. We can see the other but we cannot see ourselves. We are all here and yet at the same time none of us are here. We are made to see one another face to face. We are speaking to one another in a very subtle language, the language of sacred knowledge. We are telling the other, "I'm not really here at all."

Om Shanti.

THE EVER-WATCHFUL EYES

When you look in somebody's eyes, what do you see? Just eyes, right? What are the eyes telling you? Nothing. Absolutely nothing. Eyes do not tell you a thing. But they fix you in nonduality. They can fix you there so much, that you get scared and you run. Why? Because you are caught up with the *māya*, the illusion that is all around. The eyes themselves are living tools of sacred knowledge. They tell you nothing. The mouth tells you everything. But the eyes do not say anything. They are silent, and they are taking you to that sacred place. But you don't go there because you are scared. You get caught up in the *māya*, the body, which is what you know best. But the body is an illusion, it is changing. Anything that is changing cannot be trusted. Do not trust anything that is moving. It is changing. Let it alone. Leave it, let it pass, let it pass. Think of it as a snake. It is going by. Just let it go. Do not try to hold on to it. Let the body alone and look at the eyes.

The eyes are eternity's tools. Every pair of eyes says the same thing: nothing. And this nothing is a kind of invitation. When you look at someone you feel that nonduality. But then you look at the smile, and you look at the walk and you get stuck in the body. But go to the soul of things instead. And there, there is nonduality, perfect peace. Nonetheless, you have to live with the body. Know this and then use the body for the perfection of this realm: the world of cause and effect. Let this be your duty in life. Our goal is to perfect the imperfections of life. There are many imperfections in life. Why? Because we have to work toward perfection. If everything were perfect, there would be nothing to do. We would die. The imperfections give us purpose.

Do not look at a body and call it beautiful or ugly or skinny or fat. It is just a body, and it is changing, moving. Enjoy it for the moment but know it will eventually die. It will disappear. So don't be trapped.

The eyes are very sacred. They are still. They do not say anything. Every pair of eyes you look into says the same thing, no matter what eyes you look at. Look into the cat's eyes, into the dog's eyes, into any pair of eyes. They say the same thing. I have two beautiful dogs. Sometimes their bodies are pleasing to look at. But then I look into their eyes. It is the same as looking into your eyes. It is the same thing. No difference. The eyes do not say anything. They are falling into eternity, falling into that sacred place. According to the *Ṛg Veda*, *puruṣa* (pure consciousness) has a thousand eyes. Wherever you look those thousand eyes are looking at you. The eyes are everywhere, thousands upon thousands of eyes. And yet the drama, the world of cause and effect, continues. The movement is something you have to get in tune with. Then it is beautiful.

Om Shanti.

TRANSFORMATION: BODY, MIND AND HEART

We have to allow ourselves to be transformed. In Yoga, transformation does not come about because it is the polite thing to do or the correct thing to do. The Yogi does not live with those ideas in mind. The Yogi lives with Yogic intentionality, through the *yamās* (abstinences) and *niyamās* (observances).The *yamās* are nonviolence (*ahiṃsā*), truthfulness (*satya*), nonstealing (*asteya*), continence (*bramacarya*), and nonpossession (*aparigraha*). The *niyamās* are purity (*śauca*), contentment (*saṇtoṣa*), austerity (*tapas*), self-study (*svādhyāya*) and devotion to the Lord/Vision (*Īśvara praṇidhāna*). Each of these is part of your structure as a human being. It is already in you to live nonviolently. You do not want to hurt anyone; you want to be in harmony with nature. Is it not already the case? A Yogi must make this visible, make manifest the unmanifest.

For the Yogi, the way one lives, the way one talks, the way one is are all manifestations of transformative intentions. We live in the manifest world, and therefore we have to make manifest who we want to be. Each moment allows us to be transformed. This moment, the *ṛtu* (moment of sacrifice), allows us to manifest the world. This space is provided for us to present ourselves. The moment is waiting for us to show our intentions. Despite all the *saṃskārās*, all the past impressions, a Yogi lives with Yogic intentions. To do this, one has to be of service, be caring, be loving, be generous, be patient, be strong.

There is much confusion in the world, but to the Yogi all this can be overcome. The Yogi delights in the *atman* (the Self), in the present, upholding all life as the Self. The Yogi realizes that there are cultural differences, problems in societies, family problems, problems with friends and neighbors, problems on the job. But the Yogi lives in the light, knowing that he or she is beyond the body, beyond the mind. Through everyday living, the Yogi overcomes any obstacles in the moment. A Yogi never runs from anything. If you run from something, you are running away from the Self. You cannot run from the Self because everything is the Self. So what can you run from? Only from confusion and ignorance. Once you understand the confusion, there is no more running. There is just standing, sitting or waiting to overcome. Let all the problems come and you will overcome them. Do not avoid them; the sooner you work them out the better off you are.

We all can overcome obstacles. In childhood you overcame many obstacles, even minor ones such as not wanting to go to school. Now in adulthood you have adult obstacles and you have to overcome them. Obstacles must go, because the Self is pure. Why? Because you are *satyam* (truth), you are born pure. The confusion you feel is the confusion of the mind. But you are very pure and anything pure cannot be defiled. Your true Self can commit no falsehood, because there is nothing false about your true Self.

You have to change your body through the mind. The mind and the body have to work in harmony with each other. The mind has to create a new body, and the body has to uphold a new mind. Confusion is of the mind. You will not eat from a dirty plate or drink from a dirty glass. Your body will not allow it. You will not eat food that has been left out for four days. Your body will not let you put on clothes that are soiled and dirty. Why not? Because you are *satyam*, because you are truth, because you are clean. It is not merely because you are conditioned to wear clean clothes. Even if you were not conditioned, you would not eat anything inedible. There is a purity about you, and that you must honor. You cannot expect someone else to honor that. You will have to honor that purity yourself, by the way you live, the way you talk, by the way you are.

You are a life that is being supported by life, and therefore it is your responsibility to support life. This is accomplished by being of service, by never saying that you are tired even if you feel tired. If you are tired, take a break, sit down for a few seconds, and the pain will go away. If you are thirsty, take a drink of water. Never say in frustration that you are tired of doing something. That is not the case; the Self never tires. It is the mind that is attached, the mind that is greedy, the mind that is contaminated by the *kleśās*. It is the mind that will say "I am disgusted." Feel it in the body but avoid saying it. Let the body work it out. Let the mind live Yogic intentions, and the body will work it out. The body is in service and knows how to work it out. The body is full of service. The body is of the moment, of the *ṛtu*. The body is made to serve. The mind has to know this and the mind must liberate the body to do what must be done. When the mind has negativities such as greed, lust and egoism, then the body becomes distorted. The body shakes, the body quivers, the body sweats. The mind must release the body to just be.

The mind is always grabbing us, taking us away from this divinely-structured life. The conditioned mind judges the rights and wrongs. The conditioned mind says, "If I eat too much I'm a glutton." Remember, you are not feeding the mind, you are feeding the senses. There comes a time when the senses say they have had enough. But later they will go back for more because that is what the senses live for. They live through the consumption of all kinds of delights. But you can only eat a bit of it. You cannot eat too much. You are not really eating; you are only feeding the senses. If you ever get to that point where *you* are not the doer, you will live a very healthy, fulfilled life. Let the senses enjoy, but do not claim the enjoyment.

Consider the heart. The heart has been subjected to indifference, ingratitude and suffering. The heart has learned to die and not live. The heart must become empty. Only then can compassion, affection and caring live again. Learn once again to think with the heart and give from the heart, no matter how many abuses you have suffered. Do not hide the heart away like a turtle that pulls in its head for fear of being trampled. Only a heart that knows pain can sing, only a heart that knows pain can care. Every noble sage, every great being has suffered. Open the heart and offer yourself this day and every day.

This is the *kurukṣetra*, the battlefield of life. Remember the challenges that must be conquered. Remember Arjuna who had to fight the obstacles each day. Live in your heart, think with your mind, serve through your body. Discrimination is of the mind, living is from the heart. If one door closes, another will open. Keep the heart open. You must be, you must cry, you must laugh, you must live this life. Taste of it and be filled with it. The only reason the heart becomes constrained is because there is attachment to all the obstacles, all the fear and all the greed. Overcome these. To liberate the heart is the greatest challenge of being human. Spread your heart out. It will not be hurt; it is very strong. The whole world is in it: the sky, the ocean, all living beings, all things you fear, and all things you love. All is in the heart.

Om Shanti.

MEDITATION EXERCISE: FIXING THE MIND

Breathe in and hold.
Breathe out.
Breathe in and hold.
Breathe out.
Breathe rapidly.

Keep your eyes closed.
Focus your attention
in between your eyebrows.

Breathe in and hold.
Breathe out.
Breathe in and hold.
Breathe out.
Breathe in and hold.
Breathe out.
Breathe rapidly again.
Breathe in gently and hold.
Expel and hold the exhalation.
Breathe in and hold.
Expel.
Breathe in and hold.
Expel.
Remain exhaled.
Release.
Focus in between your eyebrows,
at the seat of intuition.
(This portion of the exercise is repeated.)

Slowly open your eyes
and look at the floor in front of you.
This is the practice of *dhāraṇā* (concentration).

*Deśa-bandhaś-cittasya dhāraṇā.**
(Concentration of the mind is [its] bondage to a place.)
Fixing the mind on one place,

on one object for a prolonged time
will eventually lead into meditation (*dhyāna*)
which is a prolonged state of concentration.

Close your eyes and look.
Open your eyes and look at the same spot
in front of you on the ground.
Breathe normally and feel comfortable.
Keep the breath at a pleasant rhythm.
Pick your head up and look at an object
on the *havan* (altar).
Continue the practice of *dhāraṇā.*

Deśa-bandhaś-cittasya dhāraṇā.
The mind has to be fixed
because the mind is restless.
It moves from circumstance to circumstance
and from object to object.
Keep the back straight and the body erect.

Sthira-sukham āsanam .**
(*Āsana* is steadiness and ease.)
The body must be firm and steady.
It must be comfortable in order to go
into *dhāraṇā*, into *dhyānam*, into *samādhi.*
Keep watching the object of your intention.
When the process of meditation gets
deeper and deeper, all else disappears.
This mind has to be steady
in order to eventually reach *nirodhaḥ.*
To the Yogi, this is a must.

Om, Shanti, Shanti, Shanti.

* *Yoga Sutra* III.1
** *Yoga Sutra* II.46

THE PRESENCE OF THE PRESENT

Within the present there is the *presence*. We are looking for the changeless in the change. Many faces, many bodies continually moving around us, but the presence of the *other* is always the same. Know that and be free. There is a special feeling of closeness when we experience that presence. It does not matter what it is. The presence is divine. I cannot even begin to communicate how precious it is.

There are extraordinary practices to help you realize the presence of this present moment. In the presence of the present you are whatever is in front of you. Every negative or positive thought just disappears in that presence. You have no thoughts then. Of all the trips people talk about, this is the greatest one. The deeper you go into it, the more you will know it in your daily life. You will be amazed at what you begin to experience. In that moment you cannot think, you cannot even name it. In the presence there is no name. This is Yoga. In that moment there is no thing, no suffering; just the contact, the presence.

With much practice we will enter the realm of the presence and begin to feel ecstasy, a whole body sensation. It is like a male/female embrace and resembles sexual bliss. However, physical bliss is the human level of ecstasy. The individual must go beyond conventional experience to attain that elated ecstasy which is of a divine nature and never changes. It is in everything, everywhere, every individual. The ignorant are afraid to make this contact because they do not know what to do with it. Hence, Yoga *sādhana* (Yoga practice) is very important.

We always have the present and that is all we have. This is a fact, a reality. Do not think "Oh, I don't have it, I don't think I can." Live in such a way that others can live through you. Give to others, but do not let them abuse you. Separate the mere taker from that one who needs to live. A child needs to live, so you can give without question to a child. Living so that you can give to the other is sacrifice. It is a very beautiful place, though it is a hard place to live in. But once you bring it to mind all the time, then there is only the moment, only the now, only the present. You will be provided with wealth, understanding and knowledge. All will be provided in the moment so that others may live through you. It will come automatically when the moment is respected.

Be brave in life. Be strong. Do not feel any guilt. What was, was. The past is a dream. The future is yet to be. The present is the perfect time. In the present there is only the presence. Do you know what that means? I adore the presence of you. The presence of a flower opens up the fragrances in my life, brings out the subtleties, the quietness, the gentleness, the presence.

In the present we have the presence. Yet, instead of taking joy in this, we look for presents--the gifts. We fail to remember that we only have the present. Instead of getting into the present, we think, "What is she going to give me? What am I going to get?" But forget about the presents. Look at the individual before you; you become overwhelmed by the presence. You need not know the other person. Just look, do not stare. There is so much to look at.

If you invite a friend over for dinner, what is more important, the dinner or the friend? The visit is food in itself. It satisfies the soul and the heart. But sometimes you are so involved in the cooking and the concern for how things will turn out that the joy is killed, it dies. But the presence is still there. Even when you go to the grocery store, look at all those fruits there, look at all those colors. Look at the presence of those apples. Do not rely on your conditioned habit of consuming. Do not be a constant consumer. Our purpose in life is not to consume, but we have become consumers. We have been conditioned to do this, but it is not our nature. Our nature is to give our lives so that others may live through us. Delight in the presence of food. It satisfies you. You do not even have to eat much of it. That is why sages and Yogis eat very little. They constantly enjoy the presence. It satisfies.

We have made the mistake in life of consuming. Use fuel sparingly. Take what you need to survive, so that others can live through you. Take in such a way as the tree takes. In the moment you have everything that is needed. It only happens in the moment, the present. The moment does not happen yesterday; yesterday is gone. It is not going to happen tomorrow; tomorrow never comes. Live in the moment.

People in relationship, like girlfriend and boyfriend, are captive in the presence. The male/female relationship is so beautiful. The presence is the thing that one is connected with. But that presence is swallowed up, consumed. It should never be consumed. Once consumed, it dies. You try to get that presence back, but you have a hard time doing it. The next thing you know, you have to end the relationship and call a lawyer. There is no other way out.

Consider the beauty of the apple, the presence of the apple. Once you eat it, what happens? It disappears; you digest it. But the apple is meant to be eaten. Eaten and then remembered. How many people know what the apple really is? Many people eat "a-p-p-l-e-s," they eat the word, the letters of the alphabet. To really eat an apple you have to experience the presence of the apple, the body of the apple, the nature of that fruit. And then it is not an apple any more. It has a special name, a name that is born from within you, a name that you will give in your own special way. It is like when you give pet names to your friends or loved ones. Like that, the fruit that you eat will also be given a special meaning and it will come through you. The presence of the present is overpowering. Because we forget to remember that there is only the present-- that the past is just a dream and the future is yet to be -- we lose the presence of the present.

Om Shanti.

ALIENATION

It is so difficult for one to live a spiritual life while feeling alienated from everyone. The practitioner of the Yogic way of life seeks communion in circumstance. See the body of the divine, the many bodies around us. These must be worshipped and then given up in order to have that ultimate union. As long as you are feeling alienated in circumstance, alienated from your friends, relatives, neighbors, everything around you, it is very difficult to have a spiritual life. So look at the person next to you and ask the question, "Why do I feel so far and yet so close?" One cause of alienation lies in cultural lifestyles, the other in the *guṇās* (three attributes of experience: light, activity, and inertia). In regard to the latter, alienation is a natural phenomenon. The *guṇās* make up our particular and solitary experience-- its arising, sustaining, and falling away. Through the process of the *guṇās* we are ever in the state of becoming, and in our experience of becoming we are alone. So we must use the mind to overcome the alienation, and unite with that unity we are all seeking, the unity beyond the *guṇās*.

It is so beautiful to move the body, the physical form. It is very important to do so. Move this body. This body only knows pain. I can tell you from experience! *Dehe, dehe, jano duhkho, mon tu me, ānando thakho*. (This body, this body, knows only pain; but You, O Self, remain in bliss.) There is the body. There is the mind. And there is the *ātman* (the Self) . The body can be used and it can be abused. But the mind and the *ātman* are something else. Where is your body? What has it done? Where is your mind? Have you made contact with the Self?

In life we are all moving to become. You are moved according to your needs, according to your desire, according to your mind. Where you put your thoughts, you become that. But what is the right purpose, the proper way, the true course to take?

One may be conditioned to seek a spiritual life, and so one learns to do so. There are so many ways of seeking a spiritual life. But the one who desires the ultimate does so not because he or she is trained to live a spiritual life, not because he or she is told to, or externally stimulated to do so. Such a one desires the spiritual life because he or she hears the inner call. The hearing must become acute, and one hears the call.

Do you spend enough time meditating to hear that call? The *ātman* (Self) wants to be released, to become united with the *paramātma* (the absolute, the totality). The physical life in this body goes through many changes. And yet there is the other, the other that never tires, never goes to sleep, never takes a vacation. Like the breath, it is always there. The mind wanders aimlessly; forget it. Seek the spiritual in you. Seek it even though the body begins to go astray, even though circumstances change. Friends, relatives, and circumstances constantly change. Remember the one within you that changes not.

Cultural alienation is also felt: the conditioned separation and distance between one human being and another. Even though two people can be sitting and eating together, they are miles and miles away, thousands and thousands of miles apart. This can be changed. Even the situations in which countries and nations are still arguing can be changed. All the conflict is nonsense and sustains alienation for, at heart, every human being all over the world is calling out for the *One* ; yet they seem so separate.

It is like a family. There is one father and one mother, and yet all the children may grow up feeling alienated from each other. A mother may have many children, but the child has only one mother. A father may have many children, but the child only has one father. Each one is calling out to mother, calling out to father. In a family you can find several children, and when they grow up each one will have great difficulty recalling experiences that they had together in the family. Surprisingly, they ask one another, "Oh, you did that? I don't remember you doing that!" They do not see the family as a unity.

Alienation in this society is felt very strongly because there is no joint family custom where one lives for the other, and all live for the *dharma* (law, righteousness). In India the practice of Yoga helps the individual realize detachment from the tight-knit family system so he or she can seek Self-realization. Yoga is a form of divine alienation. But in the U.S.A., in this nation of alienation, the family does not begin in unity. In many cases there is little or no honor given to father or mother. The plan of the society seems to remove the child from mother and father. The child spends long hours at school and many hours watching television. In many homes both parents are away at work most of the day. Of course, each child, each of us individually, knows we love our parents. We know that. But the respect has been very slowly eliminated. Children at a very early age, as early as ten, go out of the house and do not care what mother or father says.

The absence of nurturing has caused alienation among people. And so the heart is dry. Love is simply put in a vault. The numbers to open up the vault cannot be found. The combinations are missing. But the love is still there. We all want to love. Everyone wants to love. I have been here and also in India, and I can see the forces of life that have brought about these conditions. I am sad that alienation is experienced.

Alienation. How do you cure this? Do not look for bigger houses and more rooms. Do not look for more. Look for each other. See what you have in front of you. It is very difficult to see what you have, because you will see what you have in accordance with your conditioning, and this conditioning will tell you that you don't have enough. Become more diligent in your looking and try to break the barriers of alienation. Seek that pure part of you so that you can see it in each living being.

Om Shanti.

BEYOND THE BEYOND

We are here in this place that never ends. It always is. We must let the light in. We must see the light in our life. We must be able to touch it. We must be able to feel it.

Being on the Yoga path takes a love that never ends, not a love that stimulates us into just being compassionate or being very nice or feeling good. It is a love beyond all that. You were born out of that love. It takes love to stay on the Yoga path. The Yoga path is not dogmatic. It is very real. It does not say that you are a good person or a bad person. It does not say this is right, this is wrong. There are no judgments. Therefore, all are called to be perfect.

Everyone is looking for a place to be in. Give me a place. Give me a name. What place? What name? And how am I to act in this place? All those that you see have positions, but with the positions come many dispositions. The human being is restless in this world of duality and works endlessly toward perfection. What is perfection? The human being tries to find out. What is it? One can say, "For me it is this." Another will say, "But for me it is that." Well, what is *this* and what is *that* ? This I would like to know! You find yourself parched in the throat, your tongue sticking to the roof of your mouth for the want of the perfect word. What is perfect? What is truth according to history? According to traditional language? According to cultural embodiments? The human being is expected to find the truth.

We go from book to book, from movie to movie, from human being to human being, from one extreme to another looking for that surprise package, looking for the *this* or *that*. It is beyond the body, beyond the mind, beyond the senses. Can you go beyond that? Do you have the love to go beyond that? It is not that. It is not me. What is it? I cannot see it. Where is it? I cannot hear it. How is it? I cannot speak it. Then what is it? You might say, "Oh, yes, it must be something that you can't see." And so we go on with this type of thinking. We go after something that we cannot see with the desire to see what we cannot see. Hence, we go on looking for *another object.*

The truth is we are born of *that* which can never be an object. We are *that* and we have to be able to know *that* in each other. People will say they are looking for love, looking for God, looking to be popular, to get very rich, to have many friends. People have so many desires. Have it all! You can have it with no problem. The world is filled with these things and you can certainly get a little piece for yourself. But it will not be enough, even if you have five million dollars. Do you know the headache that comes with five million dollars? With every negative there is a positive and with every positive there is a negative.

The duality in this human existence does not end. So what do you have to do? The wise sages say give it all up. You may reply that you cannot, because you need some of it; you want the duality. But you must give it up. You must become one hundred percent attached and one hundred percent detached. This is the real trick. Have all the money, all the popularity. Have everything and at the same time be detached from it. Some will say that this is a contradiction. How can you have it and not have it? Some know how to and some do not. Some can do it and some will not.

We come alone in this world and we go out alone. Each one must live up to one's own consciousness and own understanding. If you are seeking the truth then look for it. It is everywhere. You cannot possess it, but just like anything else, you can have it. It is all yours because you are *that.* It is an amazing thing. When you find this out, then spiritual life becomes very easy.

PLEASURE AND PAIN

In this world of cause and effect we feel many changes. We fear the changes and at the same time we look forward to the changes. We want them and do not want them. This is our dilemma. We want the summer to come and when it does we complain that it is too hot. Even after a few hours we cannot stand it.

You must have both the pleasure and the pain. You must learn to enjoy the pain. Learn to love it. Learn to like it. When it gets really hot, go into even more activity. Mop the floors clean. Do not sit and complain that it is too hot. Sweat a little more. Get the toxins out. Feel your life because that is what this life is all about. This life is for you to feel. You have to be able to enjoy the heat and the cold, the negative and the positive, the pain and the pleasure. They must be experienced and you must feel good in them. Even when you are sweating, feel good.

When people are in love and locked in an embrace, it can be very hot and sweaty. The people even stick to each other. Most of you have done that. You don't say that it is too hot then, do you? You have to find that same ecstasy when you are not in an amorous embrace. Lovemaking is twenty-four hours a day when you are locked in the embrace of the divine. It never ends. You must make the twinkle come back into your eyes and you must be constantly in love. The divine play of life must be brought into human realities. The next time you are sweating in the heat of the sun or shivering in the cold, enjoy it. It does not last long. Get into the "isness" and then it changes.

THE BLIGHT OF EGOISM (ASMITĀ)

The sense of *asmitā* (I-am-ness) is constantly present and very powerful. One must go beyond *asmitā* to realize the Self. The ignorant person does not even think about the Self because he or she is just too busy in *asmitā*. One thinks in terms of producing and sustaining and continuing *asmitā*. When one can overcome *asmitā*, one then goes beyond.

For the average person it is very difficult to know the Self, the true Self. It takes a great deal of thinking and desire. It takes passion. How can one think about higher states of consciousness when one thinks about *asmitā* all the time? One needs pain to dissolve *asmitā*. Gluttony, greed and egoism have to go. The camouflage must be removed. There is no other way.

To get rid of *asmitā*, one has to suffer. One has to bear the cross and after bearing the cross, rise again and be resurrected. Easter holds a very special message for the Christian world. Everything must be given up for the will of the Father. When Christ sacrificed everything, he left behind words of wisdom that some can understand and fully embody. Some become Christ-like. Others follow dogmatically and cannot embody the life that Christ lived. One has to fast forty days and forty nights. One has to find a garden to sit in. When one returns from that place one will feel a surge of power that is a resurrection in itself. One will be released from small-mindedness, fear and anxiety. It takes one beyond. It is an awesome responsibility.

You do not realize how much power you have. You have the power to destroy. You have the power to preserve and you also have the power to create. These are very powerful forces that you have. But when do you do it? How do you do it? Why do you do it? This day choose what you will be.

In the life of an individual, *asmitā* is a very powerful force. There are people who have reached the age of adulthood but still are children who expect everything and do not want to give anything in return. If you tell them that they are adults and they should know better, they act as if they do not know what you are talking about. They make life very miserable for others around them because they are not putting their shoulders to the wheel of life. They retard the process of evolution. These people need *tapas* (austerity, heat), work. But with the work they always want you to let them know what a good job they are doing. They want a lot of attention.

Asmitā is a destructive force when it is not surrendered in the course of everyday life. It has to be given up. It has to be used up in activity until it is swallowed up. *Asmitā* is always saying, "I'm here, I'm here, look at me, I'm here. Tell me what to do. But while you're telling me, make sure you give me flowers, too."

It takes a long time to get rid of *asmitā*. When *asmitā* is erased through activities, the movement of life is released. The individuals who have *asmitā* may be compelled to move, but they are not in the moment. It is like a car spinning its wheels but not moving. The wheels might be spinning but the car is not going anywhere. People with a lot of *asmitā* are like that. Their wheels are spinning but there is no movement. They need a little push. You have to push the car. A little pat on the shoulder, a little gesture of acknowledgment is needed by such people. They have to have it. If not, they are going to cry. They are going to bug you to death. They will not leave you alone. No matter how much you do for them, they will not accept it. It will not be enough, because though their wheels are turning, they are going nowhere. They cannot feel the motion of life.

The next time you face an individual who is stuck in *asmitā*, notice how they will carry on and tell you that you are all wrong. It is all your fault. You cannot get them to say they did anything wrong. You have to squeeze it out of them, you have to confront them and say, "Now don't you agree that was an error on your part?" But they still hold out, though eventually they may apologize.

Asmitā is no one's fault. It is not you. You are beautiful. You are divine. *Asmitā* is the energy of *saṃsāra* (cycle of births and deaths). You have to see that you are working with the energies of karmic evolution. You have to dissolve everything karmically. It takes a conscious person to do that. If you feel in a relationship that you are the more conscious one, you must watch out for your friend's *asmitā*. It comes up in those closest to you. If you are married, you have a beautiful opportunity right there, a day and night bombardment. *Asmitā* is wild and has nothing to do with the divine, the Self. It is a mixture of energies going crazy. When you meet someone who is puffed up about being a genius, you have another open field. That individual is just asking for you to sock it to them!

What happens when two individuals have strong *asmitā*? No two are in the same place at the same time. Each will have varying degrees of these negative influences. There is always one in the circumstance that will be more or less in control. Talk about the Self. Focus on the goal of life.

When you look at your friend or relative who has not reached the height of consciousness, beware. Recognize the presence of *asmitā*. Despite *asmitā*, we are searching for Self-realization. We are going toward that. In order to be Self-realized, we have to see the interplay of the *guṇās* and *saṃskārās*. We have to make the person in front of us realize that Self, not only through verbal activities but also through silent language, through gestures, through movement. Allow and encourage the changes to occur.

The most apparent part of daily living is *asmitā*. Where does that need for recognition come from? It comes from insecurity. Insecurity is grounded in ignorance regarding the true Self. When there is ignorance, there is no knowledge, no understanding. That insecurity is projected onto whatever is passing by. When one is suffering from insecurity there is no self-worth. Self-worth occurs when one is in motion, when one is turning the wheel of life. Many individuals who are supposedly practicing Yoga are just turning their own wheels. They have not even started to do *āsanās* (postures) yet. They cannot fast on a regular basis or keep silent on a regular basis. They just talk and think but are not thinking properly and are just talking at random. There is hope that at some point in time a stronger force will push and move that person. We all have to move. No one is allowed to occupy space for no purpose. What happens when a car just sits in one place? It gets towed away or ticketed. It has to move. We humans have to move too. We just cannot keep thinking and talking.

Do not think your friends and your close associates are aggravating you. This is never really the case. We are all here for each other. There is no end to all that we have. We have to begin to respect ourselves, even though someone does not respect us. Have respect for yourself. Say to yourself "I have the power to create, sustain, and destroy." You are like the trinity of the Hindu gods, Brahma, Viṣṇu, Śiva. Śiva is always sitting with his eyes closed. He is always meditating. When Śiva opens his eyes he can destroy the world; he is very powerful. The power of destruction is immense in Śiva. He sits in meditation knowing the power that he has. The three aspects of the trinity are within the individual: to create, to sustain, to destroy. Brahma, Viṣṇu, and Śiva correlate, in Yogic terms, to *sattva*, *rajas* and *tamas,* the three *guṇās*. *Tamas* destroys everything. *Rajas* preserves it. *Sattva* creates it. Look at the world around you and find your place. You have the power to destroy ignorance, to preserve the reality of life, and to worship and respect creation because that is you. You are that.

In your daily life feel the movement. Feel it. Be in it. Live through it. And let it live through you. This is life. We are a force in the world but are not of this world. Therefore we are to live for one another. We are to live through one another. Do you know what that is like? It is like the movement you feel when you walk very fast. Everything just becomes. Nothing is held back. Live through, go through another human life and let that human life go through you. Allow it to be. You need a voice of a higher command to make that happen. A voice of higher command will give you that surge of power, that strength, that courage to go through the obstacles.

Do not get emotional but be filled with motion. Motion is your life, your rhythm, your vibration. Get into the motion. You know how you feel when you walk fast. A surge of energy flows and just grabs you. Live through another body and allow that other body to live through you. It is the surrender of the mind to consciousness that allows this to be. One has to surrender to the voice of consciousness, not to the voice of *asmitā*.

When you hear someone call you, that voice is entering your body and your mind. Use your intelligence to discriminate. Is it the voice of *asmitā* or is it the voice of consciousness? How will I let this voice live through the body? What can I do with this that is entering me? Use intelligence to understand the nature of your activities. The negative and the positive are always working at the same time. This is why we have a mind to think. Think, discriminate and allow for the other to live through you and you to live through the other. Let the voice of consciousness be your guide. Seek liberation. Be at peace.

Om Shanti.

QUESTIONS AND ANSWERS

QUESTION:

What is liberation?

THE GURĀṆI REPLIES:

Liberation is accepting life. Accepting it and getting rid of egoism, *asmitā*, getting rid of the afflictions, the *kleśās*. The minute you think that you are the doer, you lose out. The minute you see yourself doing something and think, "I am doing this, I did too much," you lose out. You must never say that you did too much. You must never say that you cannot do it. Whenever the sense of *asmitā* is there, you know there is no liberation.

Doing *sādhana* (Yoga practice) is a wonderful thing. It gives you time to reflect. It helps you to recognize what is to be done to attain perfection. But it is in the karmic cycle of affairs that one knows if one is bound or free. The minute a little fear comes in, the minute a little attachment comes in, you know you are stuck, you are bound, you are not free. When there is a freedom of movement with no "me" in it you know you are liberated. There are times when you do things very freely and you feel the free movement. But what about the things you do not like to do and yet must do? That is where the challenge comes in. That is the place for you to purify yourself by saying, "I don't like to do this. I know that I am stuck but I'm going to do it." In that doing, learn to loosen up. Lighten up. Free yourself of that sticky, icky feeling that you really don't want to be doing what you must do. In that period of doing you let go, you dissolve your *asmitā*. A door opens and you walk in and you do. In the process of doing you release yourself.

Your undertakings will be in accordance with your need for liberation. Do *sādhana*, read the great scriptures, read the lives of great people. Look and listen. Use all your senses to reach into the unmanifest.

QUESTION:

How does one live a spiritual life? How can one be a Yogi? How can one get rid of the *kleśās* (afflictions, hindrances)? How can one be in the moment and give in the moment? How can one just be?

THE GURĀṆI REPLIES:

All of these are extremely difficult because we have no time to lose. We are moving. Someone is calling and we must hurry up and get there. We are running after illusion and we think that *this* will satisfy, that *this thing is It.* I have heard it all: "This woman is going to please me for life." "This man is going to be Prince Charming for all eternity." "When I get this baby, it will be the greatest thing in my life." The other popular topic is possessions: "When I buy a car...." "When I buy a house...." and "Oh, if I could get that job...." All these things are getting, getting, getting. In a sense it is fine; you have to get, you have to get before you can give it all up. You have to get it and you do get it. Just try not to get too stuck on the getting. Try to not get too attached when you get something, because when you have to give it up, it will be painful. But when that time comes, feel the pain, feel everything. This is existence and we have to feel our reality, which is suffering. Every single day you can at times identify with Christ on the cross. Every day you are crucified, even if in a small way. These are the moments we must notice.

QUESTION:

Is the desire for enlightenment a selfish desire?

THE GURĀṆI REPLIES:

It depends on the individual. The conditioned individual who is involved with constant thoughts of me and mine is selfishly looking for Self-realization, looking for another possession. But then there is the person who looks for Self-realization because all else in life has failed, all else proves false, all else is temporary. This individual seeks Self-realization because he or she knows, either directly or indirectly, that this world with all its activities is temporary. When this person seeks Self-realization it is not a selfish activity. It is a search, a crying, a movement of one's innermost feelings. After you have gone through the world with all its disappointments and you go from place to place to place, and you get disappointed wherever you go, then where else is there to go? The Bible tells of how the prodigal son comes home and says, "Father, forgive me. Father forgive me and accept me." Like that, the desire to be Self-realized is not a selfish desire, but it is a desire born out of suffering. This is a true search. On the other hand, there are people who are looking for Self-realization and it becomes another gain, another something to be done, something to be had. Then it is false activity, and one gets disappointed there too.

QUESTION:

How can I develop total concentration of focus throughout the day?

THE GURĀṆI REPLIES:

Stay in your breath. Focus comes very naturally when you have the proper intention. *Asmitā* (egoism) takes everything away. When there is no *asmitā*, the focus is very natural. Concentration and attention become perfect. Everything is perfect when there is no *asmitā*. *Asmitā* always calls for recognition. You cannot give that to yourself; only the world can give it to you. Someone can come to you and say that you did a great job. That is fine. Acknowledge praise but do not crave it. Be humble and accept that compliment because it is part of the *ṛta* (truth, norm, sacred order) to do that. Acknowledgment is fine as long as you do not blow your own horn. Do not praise yourself and say that you are doing this and that.

Concentration is a very simple thing. It is part of the flow of life, part of the *ṛta*. It is already there. It does not need to be worked at. The first thing that is needed is to surrender to life. Surrender to be wherever you are needed, doing whatever has to be done. Be a servant in life, an upholder, a caretaker. When you are there as an upholder, focus comes easy.

QUESTION:

Sometimes I do things without thinking. How can I be more conscious when I act?

THE GURĀNI RESPONDS:

There are some things that are very important to do, yet they are done automatically. You are conditioned to do those things and you do them. It is part of the day, a routine.

Doing them, even if you are not thinking about them, does not bring ill health to you and keeps you fit and healthy, like brushing your teeth. There is nothing to it. Just pay attention. But if in the moment your mind is drifting because you have no time to lose, you are in a big hurry, you want to go places and do things, then "something needs to be done." You have to slow yourself down a little and then you will be able to pay attention.

QUESTION:

What is the purpose of marriage?

THE GURĀṆI RESPONDS:

The purpose of marriage is to create for yourself a *kurukṣetra,* a battlefield. Marriage provides the ground upon which to work out one's karma. Marriage brings up tendencies for you to understand. This relationship is a divinely structured battle. Culture has made it a social act. At times, individuals will find themselves in relationships regardless of whether legal documents are involved. People live together and that also is a marriage.

With marriage there is negative and positive, as in all areas of life. Whatever you do you must do it with a free will, knowing that it is your desire to be in a relationship.

What is the purpose of marriage? It is to help see karma and how it works. Day in and day out you will be forced into action and reaction. The grind at times will be very painful and sometimes it will be filled with ecstasy. You have to think before you act. When one has true love for universal consciousness then one acts very consciously towards all living beings. There is no difference between the life of a bug and the life of a sophisticated human; both are treading upon the same path of birth and death. In the moment we live. In the moment we die. We have to be very conscious of the moment.

When spring is in the air, everyone is looking for intimacy. It is part of life, a very natural occurrence. The bees buzz around, the flowers open up. Your body is pulled into it because it is working in the rhythm of life. There is nothing wrong with that. But we humans can think and we must think. Once we take up a responsibility in life we must see it through to the end.

QUESTION:

Doing meditation and Yoga, I feel blessed with joy and fulfillment. Yet, sometimes the needs of the other start picking away at me, especially when someone says, "If you cared for me, you would do this! I need this, I need that!" It becomes so overwhelming that I am pulled away from where I should be. There are many distractions in trying to stay on the Yoga path. How does one cope when someone makes so many demands?

THE GURĀṆI RESPONDS:

Why don't you just do what is asked of you? It is much easier to just do it and get it over with than to have all that resentment and aversion. This doesn't mean that you have to do anything and everything that's asked of you. Some activities will destroy the creative process and some will sustain it. Some activities will destroy everything, including oneself. The thing to do is to remember the great powers in the world, like the wind and the sun. For instance, when the sun shines, it does not say "I will just shine on the people that take notice of me and are doing the salutation to the sun every morning. The rest can go drown in the ocean." The sun does not say that. The wind blows and blows, going here and there. It goes into everything, but never says, "I'm tired." You never hear any of the elements say, "I'm tired," or "I don't want to deal with it." Only human beings constantly complain and have an attitude. If human beings aren't complaining verbally, they have attitudes, which are just as ugly as verbal discontent. You feel those attitudes as if a bomb were hitting you. So take a lesson from the elements and be of service, just be of service constantly. Being of service is the beginning. Doing selfless service is a difficult thing for individuals who are very stuck on their preferences. They prefer to do this or that, and they prefer to do it at certain times. At certain times they will do certain things. There are many people who are stuck like that.

In the beginning it is very difficult to just surrender. There is an embodied conditioning to be overcome, so you have to be easy on yourself. Do not hate yourself for not being selfless in the moment. Forgive yourself. Be human and forgive yourself. As time goes by you will be able to be more selfless. Eventually it will become such an easy thing to do that you won't even know you are doing it. Sometimes you will be involved in action and reaction and you will not even know you are doing it. It will be done just for the sake of doing and you will be caught up in the *ṛta* (truth, norm, sacred order).

However, there are people who do take advantage of other people. You have to tell those people to not take advantage of you. Say to them, "I am your friend. I will give you a hug, I will do what you want, but do not constantly take advantage of me." Using a person in this way is an ignorant act. Only the ignorant do that. Then there are individuals who are deliberately ignorant. There are all kinds of games that people play. However, if you have a Yogic perspective all the time, no matter how dumb or how irritating an individual is, you will not let that person get the best of you. The Yogi is very powerful. A Yogi can transform another's life just by his or her actions. So your aim is not in serving and giving in to the whims of someone. The aim is to change the other. The other begins to see your actions, and will change eventually. It could take ten years, it could take ten minutes. You can never tell; that is why you keep going, and why it is helpful to think of the elements, which are timeless.

QUESTION:

Is crying a sign of weakness or is it beneficial?

THE GURĀṆI RESPONDS:

If you feel like crying, just cry- empty yourself of the heaviness you feel. Crying is an emptying. When the emotions are filled to the brim, they have to pour out, so they come out through laughter, through tears, through screaming, through yelling. The reservoir of emotions has to empty itself. In some instances, when you are full of emotion, there is nothing to do but cry. However, you must discriminate in the situation and take proper responsibility for it. If you feel any weakness coming up, forgive yourself. Do not be hard on yourself and say "I shouldn't feel this way." Sometimes this is the case: people don't want to feel what they are feeling. They don't realize that there is an aspect to a human being that is totally helpless and suffers.

However, there is another aspect of the human being that transcends suffering in the very act of suffering. In the play that exists between the two aspects we cry, laugh, sing, and dance. So do whatever comes to you as long as you are not hurting anybody, as long as you are not imposing it on anyone else. Let yourself be released.

QUESTION:

How can one use the mind to get rid of the mind?

THE GURĀṆI RESPONDS:

Where is the mind? How can you get rid of something you don't know? You have to find out what the mind is, how the mind works. Try to find out. It takes sitting, it takes exercise, it takes intentionality to bring about the understanding of what this mind is. I can take a cup and say, "This is a cup." I can show it and you can see it. What are the contents of the cup? You cannot see what is in it at this moment because the cup is up here with me. So you would have to come here and look down into the cup. Like that, you must experience and know the mind directly. Then you can get rid of it. Using the mind to get rid of the mind is a practice you have to learn. You cannot talk about it too much. You have to learn about it, you have to study.

QUESTION:

How does one achieve *citta-vṛtti-nirodhaḥ?* (Restriction of thought modifications)

THE GURĀṆI RESPONDS:

One does not achieve *citta-vṛtti-nirodhaḥ* unless one practices. One may think of it and hear many lectures about it, but it cannot be attained without practice. Do the *āsanās*. Do your *sādhana*. Honor the sages. Respect your teachers. Love one another. This is the golden rule.

QUESTION:

How can I stay in the place I find in meditation?

THE GURĀṆI RESPONDS:

Very simple. Just stay in it. Do not escape into meditation. Meditation is not to escape life. Meditation is a place you go into which makes you strong, a place beyond this world of cause and effect. Overcome the inconveniences in your life through the power you get during meditation.

Meditation is a very holy place, a very powerful place. Anyone who has been there has come out as a different person. You cannot be the same. There are reasons people do meditation, reasons people desire to be in that place. Before he was crucified, Christ went into the Garden of Gethsemane to meditate. He gained the strength to sacrifice and give it all up. According to history he was a human just like everyone else. He had the feelings and the circumstances of daily living like you and me. One must practice, must realize that this too shall pass away.

QUESTION:

How can I find peace?

THE GURĀṆI RESPONDS:

So many of life's problems lie in striving for peace. Peace is already at your disposal. You have peace. Peace is that place between the two breaths, the inhalation and the exhalation. When you feel confusion or anger, take a breath. Inhale as deep as you can, then exhale. In the exhaled breath you will experience detachment. In that space where there is no breath going in or out there is peace. In order to live with the world you find around you, understand the confusion and discriminate it away.

QUESTION:

How can I find patience? I need peace and patience.

THE GURĀṆI RESPONDS:

Patience is something you have to work at. It is the inability to sustain peace that gives you restlessness. Because you are already experiencing peace but are unable to sustain it, stress is created. What you have to do in this case is recognize from which areas in your life the restlessness is coming: people you meet, things you hear. Eliminate what you do not need. Keep the peace you have. Having peace does not mean shirking responsibility or avoiding circumstances and relationships. It means having a better understanding to cope with the realities of your life and accepting your life as it is.

We are always looking for that which we already have, because that which we already have is covered up. Hence we look for peace. We look for love. We look for friendship. These are things we already have but they are covered up. We have to remove the coverings. You have peace. You have love. You have everything.

QUESTION:

How is it that some people seem to be good, even though they do not think about it or strive for it? Can other types of people change? This bothers me.

THE GURĀṆI RESPONDS:

I am glad that it bothers you, but there is nothing you can do for someone else. You can just make sure that your own existence, your own life is lived within the *dharma* (law, righteousness). Everything will change in life. Friends will come and friends will go. People will come and people will go. But the *dharma* will not change. Because of that, uphold the *dharma*. You can bring a child up from infancy and suddenly, at age eighteen, the child says, "Good bye, Mom, I'm leaving." You have a heartache then. There is nothing you can do. You must surrender to the *ṛta*. The *ṛta* cannot do anything about it; you have to let go. You must let go of thoughts of right and wrong, of "this is good," and "that is bad." You cannot hold onto that. Yogically, from Yogic eyes, through Yogic vision, there are no rights and no wrongs.

All of life is a great happening and we must be part of that, but with detachment. Yet because we are human, we have all kinds of emotions: sorrow, hate, spite. We can become mean, treacherous and devious. All these things are due to the human reality, to just being human. There is a weakness and yet there is a strength in being human. But there is no right and no wrong. What is, *is*, and that is a fact. You have had many thoughts and great aspirations, but some things fail to be seen. We do not see what is happening because we are tired and we drift with the clouds of our mind. We just go with the thoughts. Also, we tend to want to hold onto certain ideas. We want to hold on, but this is not possible. You have to give it all up, from the smallest grain of sand to the greatest of mountains. In that moment you will have it all. In that giving up, you truly have the real thing.

The human reality is wanting things to be only "nice"; *everyone should have everything*. This is a great thought, a great human desire. But even these thoughts are culturally conditioned. There is always the desire to be perfect and the desire to have power. But the Yogi sees that there is only power; there is nothing else but power. Power creates, power sustains, power destroys. You cannot say power is right or power is wrong, power is great or power is not great. Power simply *is*.

The Yogic way of life is lived experience. Just doing the practices is not enough. Yoga is something you have to live daily; it has to become embodied. When the mind is constantly absorbed in Yoga, then you will see the power that is life. When you look at a tree, you see that some leaves on the tree are big and some are little. You will see all kinds of leaves and all kinds of trees. However, when you look through Yogic eyes, you will not see trees. All this is a great illusion, the dance of Śiva, the dance of creation.

There is the human reality, and then there also is the human tragedy. What does it mean to be human? You cry, you laugh, you sing, you dance, you feel sorrow, you feel weak, you feel strong. There are ups and downs, the changes. Physiological and spiritual changes are occurring constantly. To be human means to be constantly buffeted by changes. When are the changes going to stop? There is no end of change. You cannot stop the change. But you can achieve *citta-vṛtti-nirodhaḥ,* the state of no mind. In this state, all the mind that you have is absorbed in *Brahman*, is absorbed in the *ṛta*, is absorbed in the totality. No mind means all mind, the total embrace of the entire universe. Nonetheless, the "realities" of life will continue to be. Sitting in meditation is a temporary thing. You have to get up and take care of worldly affairs, and then all the aggravation comes up. This is part of being human.

You have to clean things up, you have to work, you have to support, you have to keep life going. It is a beautiful life. What hinders our peace, our state of *saṅtoṣa* (contentment)? It is the mind, with its preconditioned cultural values of, "I am right and you are wrong; I know what it's all about, but you do not." It is the mind that judges and says such things as, "Oh, you are two feet taller than me, I'm short and you're tall," or "I'm ugly and you're beautiful," or "Get out of my sight, I don't need you, I don't need anybody." This is conditioned, human stuckness, which gets in everyone's way. Everyone gets stuck; it's a human reality. So when you feel that you are being driven by circumstances beyond your control, when you get into a state of helplessness, think of the experience that occurs when we stand face to face. Neither I see me, nor you see you. Go into that place where there is peace. Then everything drops away and you begin to experience what is. Not what you think is, but what is.

Every obstaclc we meet in life is a challenge. Every obstacle is not a curse, is not a tragedy; it is not the end of the world. Every obstacle is a challenge, and it is a blessing. I also face obstacles. I am human too. Just because I am a Guru and have reached that ultimate state does not mean that I am past the human reality of life. When people feel sick or sorrowful or when anyone has pain or crazy circumstances, I go on the human merry-go-round. I see, feel and hear everybody's song and dance. I am seeing everything. Yes, I have reached *samādhi*. Yes, I have that superconsciousness. But then I say to myself, "You are still human, Anjali, you are still human. You can cry and you can sing and you can feel for someone. You can give all that you can give, but, Anjali, you are still human." I have to get through this human life, just like you.

Sympathize with one another, do not pick at one another. Have sympathy, have compassion. Accept the difference, accept the other. Allow for it, because you are human too. You have a long path ahead of you as a human being, so start taking control of your mind. Aim for *citta-vṛtti-nirodhaḥ*. Every time you get stuck, think of one of the Yogic teachings or think of a song or something to bring you to that point of nonduality. Duality is always full of pain, but nonduality will give you that peace that you need, the time to work out your circumstance.

Live every day as if it is your last day. Say the doctor told you you only have two days to live. Or say someone appeared in your dream and said, "Tomorrow I am coming to get you." You don't know where or you don't know how, but you know you are going to go. Your eyes will start opening very fast and become big and huge. Your hearing will become acute. You will be listening. Do not wait for such a shock. Do not wait for someone to give you that telegram. Live very actively every day, live actively with your senses. Be in tune. If you look to the side, do not waste the look. Do not look and keep your mind some place else. Remember that where the body is, the mind too must be. Be total wherever you are. Look forward. Be wherever you are. Get the full impact of wherever you are.

The light of knowledge balances off all ignorance, pierces through all suffering. May it go before you. May it be behind you. May it be beside you, this day and everyday.

ahaṃkāra - individuality, I-maker.

abhiniveśa - clinging to life, one of the five *kleśās*.

ahiṃsā - nonviolence. One of the five *yamās*.

aparigraha- non-possession, one of the five *yamās*.

āsana - Yoga posture.

asmitā - egoism, one of the five *kleśās*. Confusion between seer and seen.

asteya- non-stealing, one of the five *yamās*.

ātman- Self, *jīva-ātman*- embodied Self.

avidyā- ignorance, the *kleśa* which is the field for the others. Ignorance is seeing the non-eternal as eternal, the impure as pure, dissatisfaction as pleasure, and the non-self as Self. (YS II:5)

bhāva - state of being, mood

bindu - seed, point, origin, drop, dot, spot.

bodhisattva - one whose essence is perfect knowledge.

bramacarya - continence, one of the five *yamās*.

Brahman - the absolute.

buddhi - understanding, intellect.

citta - mind.

dhāraṇā - concentration, *ekagra-* one-pointedness.

dharma - law, righteousness.

dhyāna - meditation.

dveṣa - aversion, dwelling on dissatisfaction, one of the five *kleśās*.

guṇa - constituent of manifest world. Any of the three "strands" or primary components of experience-- *sattva* (light), *rajas* (activity) and *tamas* (inertia).

havan - altar.

jīva - being in time, an individual life.

īśvara-praṇidhāna - dedication or devotion to the "Lord," one of the five *niyamās*.

kaivalyam - perfect isolation, absolute unity.

kleśa- affliction, hindrance, misconception governing conventional experience. There are five: *avidyā, asmitā, rāga, dveṣa, abhiniveśa.*

kurukṣetra - battlefield, refers to the battlefield in the *Bhagavad Gītā.*

manas - mind-organ, conceptualizer.

mantra- instrument of thought, speech, sacred text.

māya - power of illusion.

neti-neti- not this, not that

nirodhaḥ - restraint, supression of *vṛtti* (thought).

niyama - observance.

paramātma - Highest Self.

prakṛti - Both the manifest world and its root source.

pratipakṣa-bhāvanam - cultivation of opposition (to the five afflictions).

pratiprasava - return to the origin.

puruṣa - (lit. "man") consciousness.

rāga - dwelling on pleasure, one of the five *kleśās*.

rajas - passion, activity, one of the three *guṇās*.

ṛta - truth, norm, sacred order.

ṛtu - moment of sacrifice.

sādhana - Yoga practice

samādhi - absorption, unitive attention.

saṃsāra- the wheel of existence.

saṃskāra - the living past, historical tendencies or patterns, incarnate structures.

sat - existence, truth, real.

sat-chit-ānanda - existence, consciousness, and bliss

saṅtoṣa - contentment, one of the five *niyamās*.

sattva - lightness, one of the three *guṇās*.

satyam - non-lying, one of the five *yamās*, truthfulness, authenticity.

śauca - purity, one of the five *niyamās*.

sūtra - thread, brief statement, aphorism. Used here to refer to the *Yoga Sūtrās* of Patañjali.

svādhyāya - self-study, one of the five *niyamās*.

tamas - heaviness, lethargy, inertia, one of the three *guṇās* .

tapas - (lit. "heat") austerity, bearing extremes, one of the five *niyamās*.

viveka - discernment, discrimination.

vṛtti - fluctuation of the mind, thought.

yama - restraint.

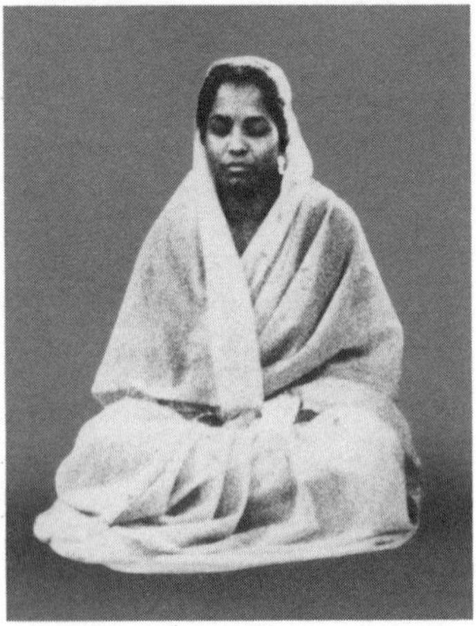

Photograph courtesy of Frances Keaveny

ABOUT THE AUTHOR

Gurāṇi Añjali* was born in Calcutta, India; educated in World Religions, Science of Āyurveda, Patañjali's Yoga, Sāṃkhya and Western Philosophy.

Having immigrated to the United States, she perceived the dire need to transmit the knowledge and practice she had embodied. Her goal then became the establishment of a center through which she could transmit what she had learned. This heartfelt desire led to the founding of Yoga Anand Ashram. The primary goal of the Ashram, since its birth in 1972, is the realization of the living goal of human existence as realized through the practice and incarnation of the Yogic perspective (*darśana*).

She lectures on all phases of life from the Yogic perspective. She is author, song writer, composer, poet and artist. Many have heard her message. She has put forth many unique Yogic exercises which lead one into a glimpse of the reality of life, the universal vision. Her book *Ways of Yoga* has also received high acclaim from many scholars and practitioners. You may contact Gurāṇi Añjali by telephone at (516) 691-8475 or by writing to Yoga Anand Ashram (mailing address) 49 Forrest Place, Amityville, NY 11701

---

* Gurāṇi is the feminine form of Guru.

ALSO AVAILABLE FROM VAJRA

Ṛtu by Gurāṇi Añjali

A book of meditational poems, each of which in its own way points to a state of unity and blessedness, experienced by the writer and made accessible to the reader through the poem.
$14.95 ISBN: 0-933989-00-8

Someone is Calling: The Songs of Gurāṇi Añjali

This audio cassette tape contains a collection of songs and instrumentals to inspire students of all spiritual paths.
$9.95

Moksha Journal

A scholarly, philosophical journal reflecting a multiplicity of spiritual perspectives, including works pertaining to Yoga, various schools of Buddhism, Sufism, mystical Christianity, etc.
$8.00 per subscription (2 issues) ISSN: 1051-127X

Twenty-Four or One by Origin

Drawing together varied musical styles: primitive, classical and contemporary, this audio cassette tape provides a tapestry of spacious melodies perfect for relaxation, meditational reflection and explorations into the realm of music, sound and rhythm.
$9.95

WANT TO KNOW MORE ABOUT CLASSICAL YOGA?

Use this form to order any of our other publications or additional copies of *Ways of Yoga*.

Please send me the following:

QTY	TITLE	PRICE *

*Please add $1.75 postage & handling for one title, $.50 for each additional title. (New York State residents please add 8½% sales tax.)

NAME: ____________________

ADDRESS: ____________________

CITY: ____________________

STATE: ________________ ZIP: ________

☐ Please add my name to the Vajra Printing & Publishing of YAA mailing list so that I may receive more information on upcoming titles.

☐ Please send information on back issues of *Moksha Journal*.

Mail to:

VAJRA PRINTING & PUBLISHING OF YAA
49-B Forrest Place
Amityville, NY 11701
(516) 691-8475